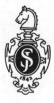

Tim Chard · Richard Lilford

Basic Sciences for
Obstetrics
and
Gynaecology

FOURTH EDITION

With 60 Figures

Springer
London Berlin Heidelberg New York
Paris Tokyo Hong Kong
Barcelona Budapest

Tim Chard, MD, FRCOG
Academic Unit of Obstetrics/Gynaecology and Reproductive Physiology,
St. Bartholomew's Hospital Medical College, West Smithfield,
London EC1A 7BE, UK

Richard Lilford, MRCOG, MRCP
Department of Obstetrics and Gynaecology, and Institute of Epidemiology
and Health Services Research, Leeds General Infirmary, Leeds LS2 9LN, UK

ISBN 3-540-19903-9 4th Edition Springer-Verlag Berlin Heidelberg New York
ISBN 0-387-19903-9 4th Edition Springer-Verlag New York Berlin Heidelberg

ISBN 3-540-19591-2 3rd Edition Springer-Verlag Berlin Heidelberg New York
ISBN 0-387-19591-2 3rd Edition Springer-Verlag New York Berlin Heidelberg

ISBN 3-540-16214-3 2nd Edition Springer-Verlag Berlin Heidelberg New York
ISBN 0-387-16214-3 2nd Edition Springer-Verlag New York Berlin Heidelberg

ISBN 3-540-12529-9 1st Edition Springer-Verlag Berlin Heidelberg New York
ISBN 0-387-12529-9 1st Edition Springer-Verlag New York Berlin Heidelberg

British Library Cataloguing in Publication Data
  Chard, T.
  Basic Sciences for Obstetrics and Gynaecology. – 4 Rev.ed
  I. Title II. Lilford, Richard J.
  618
ISBN 3-540-19903-9

Library of Congress Cataloging-in-Publication Data
Chard, T.
  Basic sciences in obstetrics and gynaecology / Tim Chard, Richard Lilford. 4th ed.
    p. cm.
  Rev. ed. of: Basic sciences for obstetrics and gynaecology. 3rd ed. 1990.
  Includes bibliographical references and index.
  ISBN 0-387-19903-9 (alk. paper). – ISBN 3-540-19903-9 (alk. paper)
  1. Medical sciences. 2. Obstetrics. 3. Gynecology. I Lilford,
Richard, 1950–   . II. Chard, T. Basic sciences for obstetrics and
gynaecology. III. Title.
  [DNLM: 1. Obstetrics. 2. Gynecology. 3. Reproduction.
4. Physiology. 5. Internal Medicine. WQ 100 C471b 1995]
R129.C44   1995
618–dc20   94–47954
DNLM/DLC   CIP
for Library of Congress   r94

First published 1983 Second Edition 1986 Third Edition 1990 Fourth Edition 1995

The use of registered names, trademarks, etc. in this publication does not imply, even
in the absence of a specific statement, that such names are exempt from the relevant
laws and regulations and therefore free for general use.

Product liability: The publisher can give no guarantee for information about drug
dosage and application thereof contained in this book. In every individual case the
respective user must check its accuracy by consulting other pharmaceutical literature.

Typeset by The Electronic Book Factory Ltd, Fife
Printed by Athenæum Press Ltd., Gateshead
28/3830–543210 Printed on acid-free paper

Preface to the Fourth Edition

In the four years since the publication of the third edition, this book has been very well received by those for whom it was intended – candidates for primary examinations in Obstetrics and Gynaecology. In consequence, we make no excuse for repeating the formula of addressing only those facts which are neither speculative nor contentious. An attempt to widen this brief would multiply the length of the book by three or four times and would place it in an identical category with several much larger texts.

As the underlying philosophy remains the same, the main changes in the fourth edition are the addition of new material and revision of existing material. Revision of existing material has been extensive with many detailed changes aimed at expanding the factual base while retaining or improving the clarity of explanation. In addition, the book is now associated with an MCQ Tutor which has proved especially popular. Finally, and probably most importantly, many of the changes are those which have been suggested by readers and reviewers of the previous editions; this feedback has been invaluable to the authors and we now hope will be equally valuable to readers of the new edition.

In this edition we wish to express our particular gratitude to Dr John Clark and Miss Lois Hague for the very elegant new illustrations in Chapter 2.

London and Leeds
July 1994

Tim Chard
Richard Lilford

Contents

Chapter 1

Cell Biology, Embryology and the Placenta

The cell

A cell consists of a nucleus, cytoplasm and a cell membrane.

The nucleus

The nucleus consists of DNA, proteins (histones and acidic proteins) and one or more nucleoli (largely made up of RNA), and a surrounding bilayer membrane which is similar in composition to the endoplasmic reticulum.

The cytoplasm

The cytoplasm contains a variety of organelles:

1. *Mitochondria*: These have inner and outer bilayer membranes. The inner membrane has numerous folds (cristae) which contain the respiratory enzymes and cytochromes of the Krebs cycle, principal energy source of the cell (via adenosine triphosphate, ATP). Mitochondria also contain self-replicating DNA. This is arranged in circles, is inherited exclusively from the mother, and codes for mitochondrial enzymes such as cytochrome oxidase and ATP synthetase.

2. *The cytoskeleton*: A system of filaments which are responsible for shape, motility and contact inhibition. Three kinds of filaments occur: microtubules (20–27 nm in diameter, which contain tubulin and are responsible for migration of chromosomes and beating of cilia and flagella); intermediate filaments (which contain tissue-specific proteins, e.g. cytokeratin in epithelial cells); and microfilaments (4–12 nm in diameter, which contain actin).

Table 1.1. The chemical composition of extracellular and intracellular fluids

	Extracellular (mEq/litre)	Intracellular (mEq/litre)
Na^+	142	10
K^+	4	140
Ca^{2+}	5	<1
Mg^{2+}	3	58
Cl^-	103	4
HCO_3^-	28	10
Protein	5	40
Glucose	5 mmol/l	0–1.7 mmol/l

3. *Lysosomes*: Packages of hydrolytic enzymes involved in phagocytosis and other 'garbage' collection functions.

4. *Ribosomes*: Granules of RNA; aggregates of ribosomes are polysomes.

5. *Endoplasmic reticulum*: A system of membranes continuous with the nuclear envelope and the cell membrane, and enclosing tubules and cisternae. The wall of the endoplasmic reticulum may be 'smooth' or 'rough', the latter bearing the ribosomes which are responsible for most protein synthesis within a cell.

6. *Golgi complex*: A group of smooth membranes enclosing cisternae. All newly synthesised proteins are directed to the Golgi complex where they are sorted for their correct intracellular destinations.

The cell membrane

The cell membrane is a bimolecular sheet of lipid molecules penetrated by islands of glycoprotein molecules. Membranes of adjacent cells may fuse (desmosomes) or communicate via channels (gap junctions) or be closely apposed as 'tight junctions'. Gap junctions contain pores which allow passage of molecules up to a molecular weight of 1500; this molecular interchange is the key to the development of the early embryo. Many epithelial cells have a surface of microvilli (1 μm in length) which increase the effective surface area; each microvillus has a core of 40 actin filaments.

Transport through the cell membrane

Differences between intra- and extracellular fluid are summarised in Table 1.1.

There are three methods by which molecules cross the cell membrane:

1. *Diffusion*. Substances which are both water and lipid soluble (oxygen, carbon dioxide, alcohol, fatty acids and certain drugs) diffuse directly across the lipid layer. Certain small molecules (e.g. water, chloride) diffuse through

membrane pores (8 Å) which are associated with the membrane proteins. In the renal collecting tubules the size of these pores is under the control of antidiuretic hormone (ADH). Many substances (e.g. glucose and galactose, but not fructose) cross the membrane rapidly by the process of 'facilitated diffusion', which is not energy dependent and involves the combination of the molecule with a carrier protein. This mechanism becomes 'saturated' at high substrate concentrations.

2. *Active transport*. This is energy dependent (using ATP) and involves combination with specific membrane-bound carrier proteins. An example is the sodium/potassium pump based on Na/K ATPase as a carrier (Fig. 1.1). A similar energy-dependent mechanism exists for monosaccharides (including fructose) and certain amino acids in intestinal epithelium and renal tubules: for sugars this is linked to the sodium pump so that both molecules follow the gradient established for sodium.

3. *Endocytosis (pinocytosis, phagocytosis)*. This is the process by which large molecules or particles are absorbed into the cells as a vesicle. Molecules first bind with the specific receptors and this triggers endocytosis. IgG crosses the placenta in this way, as do some growth factors. The endocytotic vesicle discharges its contents in the cytoplasm and is then either destroyed by lysosomes or transported back to the surface for reincorporation in the cell membrane.

Intercellular matrix

This is most abundant in connective tissue. It consists of ground substance (mucoproteins, mucopolysaccharides) and collagen fibres. Collagen is a protein with a high content of proline and hydroxyproline. Immediately after

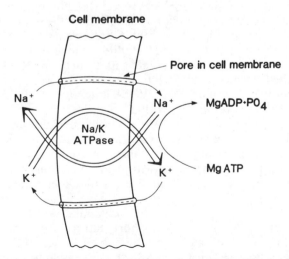

Fig. 1.1. Active transport of Na^+ and K^+ through cell membrane. The exchange of Na^+ and K^+ via the carrier protein is much more efficient than simple diffusion through pores and thus a sodium–potassium gradient is created.

secretion from fibroblasts the molecules are random and have no strength. They then become organised into 'tropocollagen', macromolecules of three chains twisted around each other in a rope-like right-handed coil. In turn, these fibrils are organised as a 'knitted' meshwork of considerable tensile strength. Collagen is of four types: I (mature collagen in dermis, bone and tendon); II (unique to cartilage); III (early scar tissue, cardiovascular tissue); IV (basement membrane, amorphous rather than helical). Cells are fixed to the matrix and to each other by a group of molecules known as integrins (e.g. laminin, fibronectin).

The genetic code

Chromosomes

The chromatin of the human nucleus is arranged as 46 chromosomes (22 pairs of autosomes and one pair of sex chromosomes, XX or XY). Each chromosome contains a double helix of deoxyribonucleic acid. The autosomes are grouped according to size, group A being the largest and group G the smallest. When the centromere is centrally placed, the chromosome is 'metacentric'; if it is off-centre, the chromosome is 'submetacentric'; and if it is near the end of one arm, it is 'acrocentric'. The chromosome adjacent to the centromere consists largely of genetically inert 'heterochromatin', which remains densely coiled during interphase (euchromatin only becomes coiled during mitosis or meiosis).

Chromosomes which are not metacentric have long (q) and short (p) arms. Chromosomes which are similar in size and shape may be distinguished by means of banding techniques with dyes such as quinacrine (Q banding) and Giemsa (G banding). G and Q banding techniques stain the same adenine–thymine rich portions of chromosomes, and a reverse technique (R banding) stains guanine–cytosine rich areas. Banding patterns show genetic polymorphism (i.e. differ between individuals) and it is sometimes possible to trace fetal autosomes to a specific parent. Chromosomes 13, 14, 15, 21 and 22 have small terminal fragments called 'satellites'. Genes (nucleolar organisers) adjacent to these satellites are translated into nucleolar RNA. These genes and the satellites are incorporated into the nucleolus during interphase. The size and shape of the satellites, and of the long arm of the Y chromosome, varies greatly between normal individuals.

In the female (XX), one of the X chromosomes exists in a tightly coiled form and, after staining with basic dyes, can be seen as the sex chromatin or Barr body. Only the terminal portion of the p arm of this chromosome remains active (the Lyon hypothesis). Inactivation of one of the X chromosomes is controlled by a specific inactivation site on the X chromosome. Thus the female carrier of an X-linked deficiency will have 50% of the normal amount of deficient substance, e.g. a carrier of haemophilia will have about 50% of the normal levels of factor VIII. The short stature of patients with Turner's syndrome is due to loss of a gene on the short (p) arm of the X, and genes on the long (q) arm are critical for ovarian development.

The Y chromosome is less than half the size of the X chromosome and can be identified by brilliant fluorescence of the outer two-thirds of the long arm

(q) after quinacrine staining. The genes for testicular formation are situated in the short arm. In 1 of 3000 people, the fluorescent heterochromatin on the Y chromosome is translocated onto an autosome and may thus be present, albeit rarely, in phenotypically normal females.

Deoxyribonucleic acid

Deoxyribonucleic acid (DNA) is a linear molecule made of bases, each of which consists of a nucleic acid (adenine, thymine, cytosine or guanine), a phosphate and a five-carbon sugar. The pentose molecules alternate with phosphate groups to form the backbone of the molecule. Carbon atom 5 of one pentose ring is connected to carbon atom 3 of the adjacent pentose by a phosphate group. This forms the 5′–3′ phosphodiesterase linkage. Nucleic acids possess polarity, in that one terminal pentose bears a phosphate group attached to its 5 carbon atom (referred to as the 5′ end), while the other terminal pentose bears a free 3-hydroxyl group (referred to as the 3′ end). The two helical polynucleotide chains have opposite polarity, i.e. they are anti-parallel, one running from the 5′ to the 3′ end and the other from the 3′ to the 5′ end.

The nucleic acids of the complementary strands form pairs: adenine–thymine and cytosine–guanine. Thus if one chain has the sequence 3′-AGGTCG-5′ the complementary chain has the sequence 5′-TCCAGC-3′. The DNA is coiled, with 10 nucleotides per turn. The coiling is usually right-handed but short segments have left-handed turns (the 'Z' form of DNA). The human haploid genome contains 2–3×10^9 base pairs but only 1% of the total DNA codes for active segments.

Of this total DNA, 5%–10% consists of thousands of identical short sequences ('highly repetitive DNA'). These are genetically inert and much of the heterochromatin and C bands are made up of these sequences. A second class of DNA is made up of sequences which are repeated from 10 to 10 000 times, and this makes up 25% of the total DNA. These 'repetitive DNA' sequences contain the genes for ribosomal RNA and the histone proteins. The remaining 65% of human DNA is termed 'unique DNA' and consists of those DNA sequences found in one to a few copies per haploid genome. This DNA contains the classic genes coding for enzymes and other polypeptides.

These active genes are separated by large segments of chromosomes, containing unique and repetitive DNA, which do not code for specific products. This DNA, interposed among the known genes, may be involved in memory or antibody formation, serving as a bank of usable code. Some of this DNA resembles that of active genes, and these portions are called 'pseudogenes'.

Within each gene, inactive segments of DNA (introns) alternate with active segments (exons). Some substances are coded by genes in completely different parts of the chromosome, e.g. the α-chain of haemoglobin is coded by two separate genes on chromosome 16.

DNA in non-bacterial (eukaryotic) cells is associated with basic proteins (histones) and acid proteins to form chromatin. The DNA strand is wound around the histones in certain areas, called nucleosomes, leaving intervening sequences devoid of basic protein (Fig. 1.2). The length of intervening

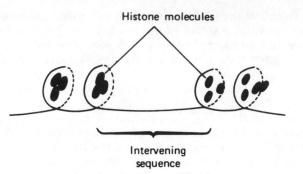

Fig. 1.2.   Relationship of DNA to histone molecules.

sequences is specific for the tissue concerned. During mitosis, dense coiling of the chromatin makes chromosomes visible to light microscopy.

Methods of DNA analysis

Many genetic diseases can now be defined at the molecular level. DNA from any cell type can be used but white blood cells are most commonly analysed. Phenol extraction and ethanol precipitation of 20 ml of blood gives 1 mg of DNA. Smaller quantities of DNA can be multiplied prior to analysis by the polymerase chain reaction (PCR).

Restriction endonucleases

Restriction endonucleases are enzymes which recognise a short nucleo-tide sequence in double-stranded DNA. They cleave the DNA molecule whenever a 'restriction site' (4–8 nucleotides) is encountered. More than 100 restriction enzymes, each with a specific restriction site, are known. Following restriction endonuclease treatment, DNA is split into multiple fragments which can be separated by gel electrophoresis. An individual gene is found on a specific fragment of DNA or, if more than one restriction site is present in the gene sequence, parts of the gene may be found on multiple fragments.

Often the cleaved DNA fragment has a 'sticky end', a single strand of DNA, which can bond to other fragments. This property is the basis for the addition of a specific DNA sequence to a microbiological vector for recombinant DNA technology.

Southern hybridisation

Following electrophoretic separation a specific DNA fragment is identified by 'Southern hybridisation' or 'Southern blot'. The DNA is denatured to create single-stranded DNA. The electrophoresis gel is blotted with nitrocellulose paper, thus transferring the DNA fragments to a solid phase. An isotopically labelled (^{32}P) probe is applied. This binds to a specific DNA fragment which can then be identified by autoradiography. The probes may be DNA, complementary mRNA, complementary DNA (cDNA) or an oligonucleotide (a 25–30 base sequence of DNA). Appropriate probes can identify a single base substitution in DNA (e.g. substitution of the codon CAT (valine) for the codon CTT (glutamic acid) in sickle cell disease).

Many genetic conditions are diagnosed with a probe to a sequence separate from that responsible for the condition under study. As the distance between the molecular probe and the mutation site decreases, the accuracy of the diagnosis increases. The most accurate diagnosis is made when an oligonucleotide or longer cDNA sequence spans the mutation site and thus specifically identifies the condition under study.

Restriction fragment length polymorphisms

Within the general population there are numerous DNA polymorphisms (normal variations in the DNA sequence between individuals). These polymorphisms are changes in the DNA base sequence. Polymorphisms occur only in non-coding sequences and hence do not alter the phenotype of the individual. These polymorphisms can be demonstrated by the use of restriction endonucleases, and are then known as RFLPs (restriction fragment length polymorphisms). Approximately one in every 100–200 base pairs in non-coding DNA represents an RFLP.

The diagnosis of a genetic disease is possible when the locus for the disease is included with a specific polymorphic DNA fragment. For example, the restriction endonuclease Hpal cleaves different size fragments from the HbS gene and the HbA gene. The 7.6 kb fragment from HbA is easily distinguished from the 13.0 kb fragment from HbS.

Recombinant DNA

In this process a DNA fragment containing the desired gene sequence is introduced into the circular DNA of a 'vector', e.g. a plasmid. The vector introduces the isolated DNA into a bacterium, which replicates its own DNA together with the newly introduced gene sequence. Once DNA replication has occurred, the bacterial clone containing the DNA fragment with the isolated gene is identified by Southern hybridisation. Using large quantities of cloned DNA, the base sequence of the fragment may be determined. Furthermore, the recombinant gene may be used for large-scale synthesis of the gene product (e.g. growth hormone, follicle stimulating hormone).

Gene function

All the chromosomes together contain about 200 000 pairs of genes. The position on the chromosome where each gene is situated is called its 'locus', so there are about 200 000 loci, each containing a gene (or rather a gene pair, as the chromosomes occur in pairs). The different forms of gene at a locus are 'alleles'. Genes on the same chromosome are 'linked'. Closely linked genes are seldom separated during meiosis. The function of genes is to replicate and transcribe.

DNA replication

At cell division DNA replicates during the S phase of the cell cycle. Replication involves disassembly of the DNA chains, replication of the DNA, and reassembly of complementary DNA strands. RNA primers are required to initiate the replication process. Replication begins at the site of attachment of chromatin loops to the matrix of the interphase nucleus. Multiple simultaneous replication sites (replicons) are required to replicate the DNA of a single chromosome. DNA polymerase is the primary enzyme for DNA replication; its activity increases during the S phase of the cell cycle and in cells undergoing the transition to the growth phase. Replication proceeds in a 5' to 3' direction. Each chromosome undergoes replication in a specific order, and homologous chromosomes replicate at the same time. Heterochromatin (genetically inactive chromatin) replicates late in the S phase, whereas euchromatin (active chromatin) replicates early in the cycle.

RNA transcription (Fig. 1.3)

The same nucleotides are present as in DNA except that the pyrimidine uracil replaces thymine, and the sugar moiety is ribose rather than deoxyribose. RNA forms a 3' to 5' single-stranded molecule linked by a phosphodiester linkage. There are five classes of RNA: (1) messenger RNA (mRNA) carries genetic information from the nuclear DNA to ribosomes; (2) heterogeneous nuclear RNA (hnRNA) is formed by the transcription of DNA and processed to form mRNA; (3) ribosomal RNA (rRNA) acts as a site for mRNA binding during protein assembly; (4) transfer RNA (tRNA) recognises specific amino acids and carries them into the growing polypeptide chain; (5) small RNA, composed of 90–300 nucleotides, is found in both the cytoplasm and the nucleus. The function of small RNA is unknown.

Human mRNA codes for a single polypeptide chain. The half-life of mRNA ranges from 1 h to 2 days. Stable mRNAs that code for proteins, which are the predominant products of a particular cell type, have longer half-lives. The concentration of specific mRNA in a cell is related to the specialised function of that cell. Only gene products expressed by the cell are represented in the mRNA. Of active genes, 90% are active in all cell types and 10% (i.e. 1000–2000) provide tissue specificity.

The mean length of mRNA excluding the poly A tail is about 2000 nucleotides. The poly A tail is at the 3' end of the molecule; it is added after transcription. All mRNAs have approximately 200 bases in the poly A tail, which aids in the attachment of the molecule to membranes. A methyl group (methyl cap) is added to the 5' end of the mRNA molecule after transcription. This protects the mRNA from enzyme degradation and aids in intracellular transport.

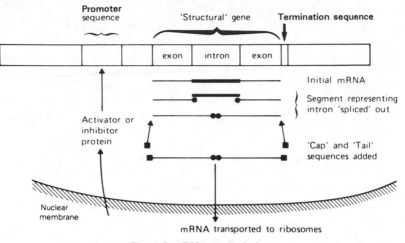

Fig. 1.3. RNA transcription.

The triplet code of mRNA determines the amino acid selected by the tRNA molecule for protein assembly. This in turn is added to the amino acid sequence of the growing polypeptide chain under mRNA direction. Selecting three out of a possible four bases gives 64 combinations. As there are only 20 amino acids, more than one triplet code may code for the same amino acid, e.g. both GGC and GGA code for glycine; mutation from GGC to GGA does not alter the amino acid sequence of the gene product.

The tRNA molecule is composed of approximately 75 nucleotides with a 3′ terminal ACC codon which attaches the carboxyl group of the specified amino acid. An enzyme (aminoacyl synthetase) attaches to each amino acid by ester bond formation to its tRNA. The anticodon loop of the tRNA has a site which specifically binds to mRNA during assembly of the polypeptide chain.

Ribosomal RNA (rRNA) forms 80%–90% of cellular RNA. It is the predominant product of transcription. The genes for rRNA are clustered on the short arms of the five acrocentric chromosomes and represent almost 1% of the coding DNA. The exact function of rRNA is unknown, but ribosomal protein synthesis does not occur in its absence.

Transcription begins at the 3′ end of the DNA molecule and progresses in a 5′ direction. Transcription of RNA occurs throughout interphase but ceases by mid-prophase of mitosis before the loss of the nucleolus and the nuclear membrane. Transcription returns during telophase. The processing of primary RNA transcripts may vary between tissues. For example, in the thyroid the product of the calcitonin gene is processed to mRNA for calcitonin, whereas in neural tissue the same gene is processed to express the calcitonin-gene related peptide (CGRP).

All cistrons have a codon for methionine, which acts as an initiator for the coding sequence of the gene. The methionine codon is then removed from the resulting mRNA. The promoter of gene expression is an adenine–thymine rich region, the so-called TATA box, which is located 25–30 bases upstream (in the 5′ direction) from the initiator site. A further 50 bases upstream the

CAT box is found. The TATA box and the CAT box are always adjacent to a specific coding sequence. At the 3' end of the molecule, an AATAA sequence indicates the end of the cistron and acts as a signal for the addition of the poly A tail to the mRNA molecule.

Every gene has either a separate regulatory gene or a regulatory sequence upstream from the cistron. Gene expression depends on both promoter and enhancer functions. The strength of the promoter is determined by upstream promoter elements (UPEs), a sequence of 8–12 nucleotides which increases the rate of transcription. Both the promoter and the enhancer interact with specific mediator proteins to increase gene expression. Some gene products (steroids and growth factors) induce their own enhancer activity.

An important controlling factor in gene expression is DNA methylation. An increase in expression occurs with a decrease in DNA methylation. The transition from embryonic to adult cells occurs with an increase in methylation, associated with a decrease in the number of mRNAs transcribed and the number of genes expressed.

Mitosis and meiosis

The cell cycle is divided into four phases: $G_1 \rightarrow S \rightarrow G_2 \rightarrow M$. M is the phase of mitosis, S the phase of nucleic acid synthesis (and DNA replication), and G_1 and G_2 are 'gap' phases. From G_1 or G_2, some cells may enter a 'resting' phase, designated as G_{0-} or G_{2-} arrest respectively. Most of the variation between cells is in G_1.

During S phase, the two DNA strands of a chromosome separate. Each strand then acts as a template for the formation of a complementary strand: the resulting double strand is thus identical with parental DNA. During prophase, the duplicated chromatin condenses into well defined chromosomes joined at the centromere, and the centrioles and their associated microtubules form the mitotic spindle. In metaphase the chromosomes assemble at the midpoint of the spindle – the metaphase plate. This is the phase at which chromosomes can be visualised for karyotyping and identified by banding. In anaphase the new sets of chromosomes separate to opposite poles of the nucleus guided by the mitotic spindle. The nucleus reforms in the telophase. Finally the cytoplasmic contents are divided (cytokinesis).

Meiosis occurs only in germ cells in the ovary and testis and involves two successive divisions. During the first stage, each of the 46 chromosomes duplicates into two chromatids, which remain attached at the centromere. They assemble side-to-side in homologous pairs, except for the X and Y chromosomes in the male, which assemble end-to-end. Cross-linkage and recombination at 'chiasmata' lead to an interchange of DNA. This does not occur between the X and Y chromosomes, which overlap end-to-end but do not pair side-by-side. The short arm of the X chromosome is involved in this partial coupling. The long arm sometimes loops back to reach the other end of the Y chromosome. The X and Y chromosomes occupy a separate site on the meiotic spindle, the 'sex chromosome vesicle'. The prophase stage of the first meiotic division is summarised in Fig. 1.4. During the second meiotic division there is no replication of DNA. In the testis the result of meiosis is the formation of four spermatids from one germ cell: each spermatid has one

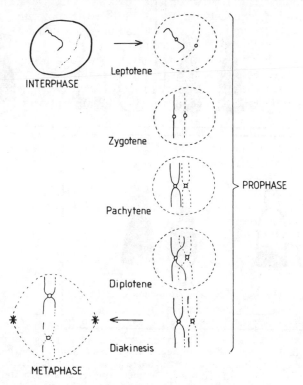

Fig. 1.4. The process of meiosis.

chromosome from each pair (haploid). In the ovary only one oocyte is formed from the two meiotic divisions. The excess genetic material is extruded as two polar bodies: one at the first meiotic division (containing 23 paired strands of DNA) and one at the second meiotic division (containing 23 single strands of DNA). The process of meiosis in the oocyte is arrested at the diplotene stage around the time of birth, and resumed just prior to the time of ovulation.

Chromosome abnormalities

Trisomy

The most common type of chromosomal abnormality is the presence of an extra chromosome – trisomy. Most trisomies are lethal, causing failure of implantation or early abortion. The three commonest surviving autosomal trisomies are trisomies 21 (Down's syndrome), 13 (Patau's syndrome) and 18 (Edward's syndrome). Even in these cases, most affected embryos abort; for example, only 20% of Down's embryos attain viability. The best known trisomy of sex chromosomes is XXY, Klinefelter's syndrome. Only one monosomy, where one of the chromosomes is absent, occurs. This is Turner's

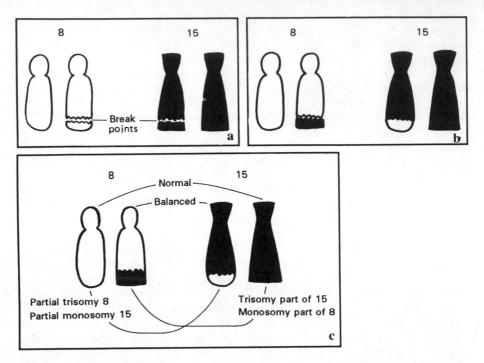

Fig. 1.5. Reciprocal translocation. **a** Breakage and **b** recombination of two chromosomes lead to this arrangement. The carrier will be normal unless a small, often undetectable, fragment of chromosomal material is lost in the process. The four arrangements which are possible in the gamete are also shown (**c**). Many unbalanced (particularly monozygotic and partially trisomic) zygotes will abort or fail to implant. Surviving unbalanced embryos will usually be abnormal.

syndrome (XO), where one of the X chromosomes is missing. This is the commonest abnormality at conception.

Mechanisms for formation of a trisomy

The most common cause of chromosomal abnormality is *non-dysjunction*; this is a failure of the relevant chromosomes to separate at meiosis, usually during the first phase. After fertilisation, the zygote has either an extra chromosome (e.g. XXY) or a missing chromosome (e.g. XO). In 80% of cases of autosomal trisomy, the causative non-dysjunction takes place in the mother, and this becomes more common with advancing maternal age. The incidence of these trisomies therefore rises with maternal age. Non-dysjunction in the father is *not* related to paternal age. In 80% of cases of Turner's syndrome the meiotic error arises in the father. The incidence of Turner's syndrome therefore decreases with advancing maternal age. Aneuploid ova and sperm are common and loss of a chromosome is more common than an additional chromosome in the secondary oocyte. Some of these are the result, not of non-dysjunction, but of anaphase lag, where a chromosome is excluded from a new cell during division. Ten per cent of sperm and nearly half of all secondary oocytes are aneuploid.

There are two other much less common mechanisms by which a trisomy may arise: mosaics and chimeras, and translocation.

A *mosaic* is an individual with cells of different chromosome constitution arising from the same zygote. This may be due to non-dysjunction during early divisions or anaphase lag. In the latter, the chromosome is delayed during its return down the nuclear spindle and does not reach the cell before the nuclear membrane closes. This gives rise to mosaicism with a normal and an abnormal cell line.

A *chimera* also has cells of separate constitution, but the two cell lines result from two zygote lineages, e.g. fertilisation of both the polar body and the ovum, which subsequently fuse, or fertilisation of two ova, which then fuse. The rare XX/XY form of gonadal dysgenesis may arise in this way.

Translocation is transfer of a segment of one chromosome to another. If the total chromosomal complement is unchanged this is harmless and described as 'balanced'. Such an individual is, however, a 'carrier'. When a break occurs in two chromosomes and the chromosome material is exchanged between the two, this translocation is said to be reciprocal (Fig. 1.5a,b). The recombinations that result from this are shown in Fig. 1.5c. If the breakage occurs at the centromere of two acrocentric chromosomes, however, the tiny short arm fragments are lost and the long arms join together; this is known as *Robertsonian translocation* or *centric fusion* (Fig. 1.6). The carrier of this translocation does not suffer any ill-effects as the short arms are in the zone of non-functioning heterochromatin. The most common Robertsonian translocation, 13/14, occurs in 1 in 1000 persons. Robertsonian translocations which can give rise to Down's syndrome include 14/21, 15/21 and 22/21. There are six possible chromosomal patterns after recombination (Fig. 1.7), three of which are immediately lethal. Theoretically, one in three of the viable offspring of such parents should be affected with a trisomy. In reality, the risk

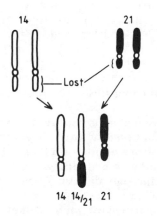

Fig. 1.6. Robertsonian translocation. Loss of the short arms and fusion of the long arms of two acrocentric chromosomes produce a balanced Robertsonian translocation with a total of 45 chromosomes.

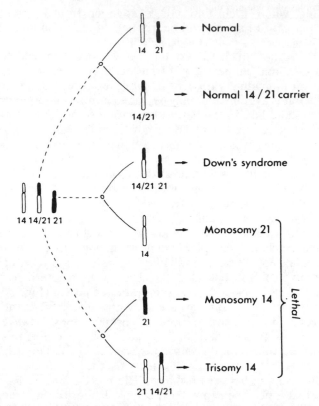

Fig. 1.7. The gametes that may result when a parent is a carrier of a balanced 14/21 Robertsonian translocation. Three of these combinations are lethal and therefore the risk of a Down's syndrome baby in an implanted pregnancy is 33%. Most of these abort and the risk at birth is around 10%.

is 10% if the mother is a carrier, as many affected embryos abort. If the father is a carrier, the risk is 5%, due to poor functional capacity of affected sperm. With the extremely rare 22/21 translocation, 100% of viable pregnancies are affected.

Other chromosomal abnormalities

Another common chromosomal abnormality is triploidy (i.e. three complete sets of chromosomes, as opposed to two). The incidence is around 1% of pregnancies; the vast majority abort, only 1 in 10 000 surviving to birth. Triploidy is often associated with hydatidiform change in the placenta. Most forms of triploidy arise through dispermy, but occasionally some follow fertilisation of a diploid ovum.

Syndromes have been described in which 'fragile' (unstable) chromosomes, which form excessive breaks in culture, are associated with clinical syndromes. In the fragile X syndrome of mental retardation these breaks occur at a specific

Table 1.2. Examples of single and multiple gene defects

Form of inheritance	Chromosome number	Condition
Dominant	4,7	Achondroplasia
		Osteogenesis imperfecta
		Most cases of von Willebrand's disease
	4	Huntington's chorea
		Marfan's syndrome
		Multiple neurofibromatosis
		Multiple polyposis
		Tuberous sclerosis
Recessive	7	Cystic fibrosis
		Phenylketonuria
	15	Tay–Sachs disease
	11	Sickle cell anaemia
	11	β-Thalassaemia major
	6	21-hydroxylase deficiency
		Galactosaemia
		Glycogen storage diseases
X-linked		Haemophilia
		Christmas disease
		Duchenne's muscular dystrophy
		Glucose-6-phosphate dehydrogenase deficiency
		Blue/green colour blindness
Multiple gene		Blood group 0/duodenal ulcer
		HLA-type B27/ankylosing spondylitis
		HLA-type DR 3 or 4/diabetes mellitus

site on the X chromosome; in ataxia telangiectasia, Fanconi's anaemia and xeroderma pigmentosum, they occur at random throughout the genome.

A rare partial deletion of chromosome 5 leads to mental deficiency – the cri du chat syndrome. Small partial deletions of chromosome 13 have been associated with congenital retinoblastoma, and of chromosome 15 with the Prader–Willi syndrome.

Genetics – single and multiple gene defects

Single gene defects

Single gene defects yield a specific abnormality and are classified, in decreasing frequency, as dominant, recessive or X-linked (see Table 1.2). The defect may arise in many different ways: (a) the gene may be totally or partially deleted (e.g. α-thalassaemia); (b) a point mutation may lead to a single amino acid substitution (e.g. sickle cell anaemia); (c) a base pair may be lost, leading to a 'frame shift' (subsequent codons are misread); (d) defects may arise at an intron–exon junction (leading to a missing or an inappropriate splice site); (e) the chain may terminate prematurely.

In a dominant defect a single abnormal gene on one of a pair of autosomes (i.e. a heterozygote) is sufficient to cause the disease. The incidence in the offspring with one affected parent is 1 in 2. If a dominant condition affects fertility it is more likely to arise by a new mutation than by direct inheritance. Thus, only 4% of cases of Huntington's chorea, which affects individuals after their peak reproductive age, are due to a new mutation, whereas 96% of cases of tuberous sclerosis, which is often lethal at an early age, are due to a mutant sperm or ovum. Many dominant conditions have incomplete penetrance, e.g. neurofibromatosis (von Recklinghausen's disease).

In a recessive defect the same gene must be abnormal on both of a pair of autosomes (i.e. a homozygote) to cause the disease. For the disease to occur, both parents must be heterozygotes; the incidence in their offspring is 1 in 4.

If a recessive mutant gene is on an X chromosome, the disease is apparent only in males (in females the abnormal X is balanced by a normal X). The risk to a heterozygous female is 1 in 2 that her son or daughter will also be a heterozygote. A female may have a sex-linked recessive disorder under the following circumstances:

1. Turner's syndrome (the X is unbalanced)
2. The mother is a carrier and the father is affected
3. The father produces a mutant sperm and the mother is a carrier
4. The patient is a phenotypic female with a male chromosome constitution (testicular feminising syndrome)

Sex-linked dominant conditions are very rare. An example is congenital hypophosphataemic rickets: here half the daughters and half the sons will be affected because the disease is manifest even in the heterozygous state. Y-linked conditions are exceedingly rare.

Multiple gene defects

Multiple gene defects are less well defined and include the increased risk of certain diseases in people with certain blood groups or histocompatibility (HLA) types. A number of genes and environmental factors combine to bring about the disease. An example is CR4 HLA type and slow 'acetylation'; in these subjects hydralazine produces a lupus erythematosus-like syndrome.

Most of the multisystem abnormalities such as cleft lip and palate and neural tube defects arise in this way, but the predisposing genetic and environmental factors are less clearly defined. Once a first-line relative has been affected with one of these conditions the chance of recurrence is about 1 in 20.

Fertilisation (Fig. 1.8)

Spermatozoa ascend the female reproductive tract largely independent of their own mobility and may be found in the ampulla of the tube only 3 h after intercourse. Only small numbers reach the ampulla where fertilisation occurs.

Two changes occur before spermatozoa are able to fertilise the ovum. The

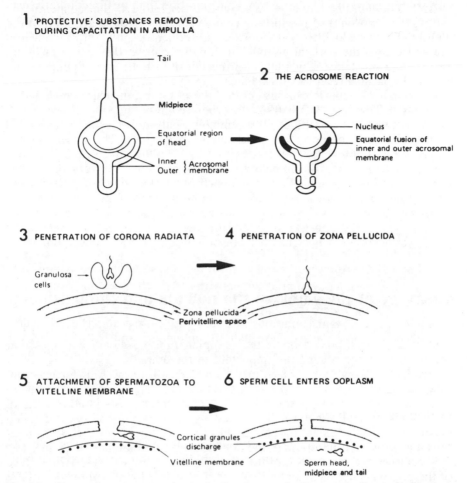

Fig. 1.8. Stages of sperm maturation in the female reproductive tract leading to fertilisation.

first change is capacitation. This takes place in the fallopian tube and takes 5–6 h. There are no obvious morphological changes, but there is an increase in motility. The life span of the spermatozoa is greatly reduced (to about 18 h). The cell membrane overlying the acrosome is depolarised and calcium enters the cell. Substances in the lower genital tract of both males and females inhibit capacitation.

The acrosome reaction begins with a swelling of the acrosome. Multiple areas of fusion then appear between the plasma and outer acrosomal membranes. Gaps develop where the membranes have fused, and the latter finally disappear altogether.

Hyaluronidase and proteinase enzymes exposed during the acrosome reaction enable the sperm to penetrate the corona radiata of the oocyte. The sperm attaches to receptors on the zona pellucida. A trypsin-like acrosomal enzyme called acrosin is then activated and enables spermatozoa to penetrate the zona pellucida to reach the perivitelline space.

After a brief interval, one sperm attaches to receptors on the cell membrane (vitelline membrane) of the secondary oocyte, causing depolarisation of the membrane (fast block to polyspermy). Subsequently, entry of calcium into the cell causes the cortical granules to move closer to the cell surface and discharge a substance which changes the density of the zona pellucida and masks the surface receptors (late block to polyspermy).

As soon as the sperm cell has entered the ooplasm, meiosis is resumed in the oocyte. This results in extrusion of the second polar body which, unlike the first, contains no granules. The remaining chromosomes are surrounded by a nuclear membrane to form the female pronucleus. The sperm nucleus enlarges within a few hours of fertilisation to form the male pronucleus; this is slightly larger than the female pronucleus and contains very prominent nucleoli. The two pronuclei approach each other (karyogamy). The nuclear membranes break down and the two gametes fuse (syngamy), with the pairing of homologous chromosomes. The first mitotic division begins. Initial development of the embryo is directed from the cytoplasm; replacement of the pronuclei by an adult nucleus does not preclude embryonic development.

Cleavage of the embryo: the morula and the blastocyst

The ovum is transported down the fallopian tube by ciliary and muscular action, the former being more important in the ampulla.

The first cleavage takes place in the ampulla within 30 h of fertilisation. The second division occurs at right angles to the first. Division occurs every 12 h and is synchronous (i.e. division occurs simultaneously in all cells) until the 16-cell stage. Daughter cells formed by the cleaving embryo are called blastomeres. They remain totipotent (i.e. can develop in any direction) until the 8-cell stage. Until the end of the first cleavage, development is directed by RNA transcribed from DNA of the oocyte. After the 8-cell stage the surface of the cells has microvilli, and cellular organelles are found at the apex of the cells. This subcellular distribution of organelles precedes differentiation in the embryo as a whole.

The embryo enters the uterine cavity at the 8-cell stage and further division results in a 16- and then a 32-cell morula. The outer cells of the morula become tightly adherent to each other with the formation of desmosomes and gap junctions (compaction). Fluid collects between this layer and the deeper blastomeres, thus forming the blastocyst. The blastocyst consists of an outer layer which will form the trophoblast, the blastocoelic fluid and an inner cell mass (Fig. 1.9). The total size of the blastocyst is the same as that of the secondary oocyte (about 100 μm in diameter), and it remains encased within the zona pellucida until shortly before implantation. The trophoblast is divided into mural and polar areas (Fig. 1.9). The latter is in contact with the inner cell mass, and new trophoblast cells are generated from this area. In contrast to the postimplantation embryo, the preimplantation morula and blastocyst are very resistant to teratogenic agents such as radiation and chemicals, which either have no effect or are immediately lethal. As the embryo enlarges from the 2-cell stage the mitochondria enlarge and develop more internal folds.

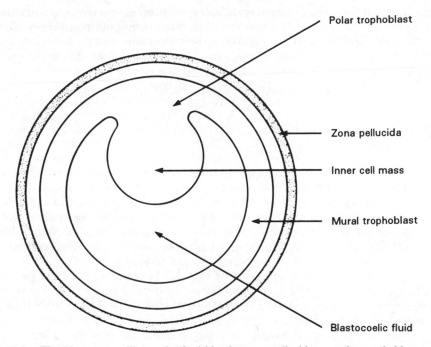

Polar trophoblast

Zona pellucida

Inner cell mass

Mural trophoblast

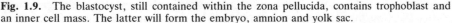

Blastocoelic fluid

Fig. 1.9. The blastocyst, still contained within the zona pellucida, contains trophoblast and an inner cell mass. The latter will form the embryo, amnion and yolk sac.

Numerous microvilli appear on the surface, but the endoplasmic reticulum does not become prominent until the 16-cell stage, when protein synthesis increases.

Oxygen consumption is low until the 8-cell stage, when the metabolic rate increases rapidly. Pyruvate rather than glucose is the principal energy substrate. The sex chromosomes (XX) of female fetuses remain active until the blastocyst stage. One of them then becomes inactive in a highly condensed form – the Barr body.

Implantation of the blastocyst and early development of the placenta and embryo

After 2 or 3 days in the uterine lumen, implantation begins. Implantation has three stages:

1. *Apposition*: The polar trophoblast comes into contact with the endometrium. Under the influence of a trypsin-like enzyme from the blastocyst the endometrium increases mitosis and produces pinopods (protrusions from

the endometrial surface) which withdraw fluid from the lumen by pinocytosis. As apposition is completed, the microvilli of both trophoblast and endometrial surface interdigitate and the pinopods are withdrawn.

2. *Adhesion*: The microvilli disappear and production of 'sticky' glyco-proteins leads to contact over a large surface area.

3. *Penetration*: Contraction of microfilaments in the trophoblast permits the blastocyst to migrate between endometrial cells. At the same time a syncytiotrophoblast forms and synthesis of trophoblast-specific proteins (e.g. SP1 and hCG) begins. Decidual cells form in the endometrial stroma. These are large cells rich in glycogen and lipid.

The trophoblast forms outer syncytial and inner cellular layers and the embryonic disc forms ectodermal (epiblast) and endodermal layers. The endoderm gives rise to cells that migrate onto the inner layer of the mural trophoblast, the two layers forming *Hauser's membrane*. The amniotic cavity forms between the cytotrophoblast and the epithelial layer of the embryonic disc (Fig. 1.10).

At 11 days Hauser's membrane acquires an intermediate layer of mesoderm. The blastocoelic cavity is now called the primary yolk sac (Fig. 1.11). The secondary yolk forms by 'collapse' of the endodermal lining of the primary yolk sac (Fig. 1.12). The 'extra-embryonic coelom' forms in the site of the primary yolk sac and surrounds the yolk sac, embryonic disc and amnion. A layer of mesoderm separates the endoderm of the extra-embryonic coelom from the underlying structures. The mesoderm between the amnion and trophoblast is called the *embryonic stalk*, which will form the umbilical cord.

At the time of the first missed period the embryonic disc is still bilaminar

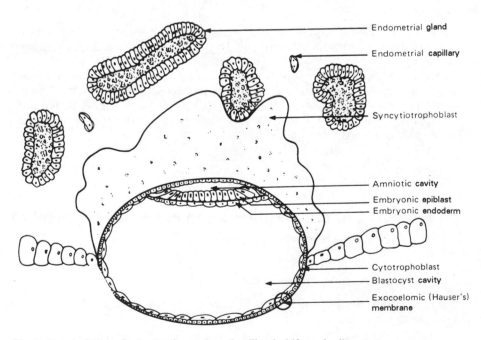

Endometrial **gland**

Endometrial **capillary**

Syncytiotrophoblast

Amniotic **cavity**

Embryonic **epiblast**
Embryonic **endoderm**

Cytotrophoblast
Blastocyst **cavity**

Exocoelomic (Hauser's)
membrane

Fig. 1.10. At 8 days the implanting embryo is still only 140 μm in diameter.

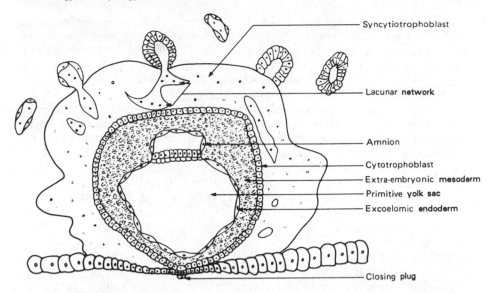

Fig. 1.11. At 10 days lacunae form and communicate with maternal blood vessels; the extra-embryonic mesoderm has started to form.

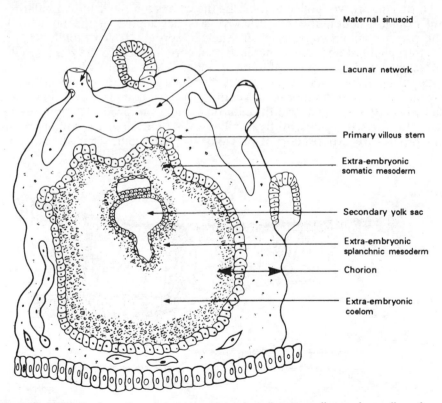

Fig. 1.12. With the formation of an extra-embryonic coelom, a small secondary yolk sac forms from the primary yolk sac. The trophoblast and mesoderm together form the chorion.

but a node of epithelial cells, the primitive streak, is forming at the caudal end. It is only 0.5 mm in size, but by this stage the placenta and membranes have undergone extensive development. The spatial identity of cells during embryogenesis appears to be directed by a group of 'homeotic' genes, which have in common a sequence of DNA referred to as the 'homeobox'.

Before implantation is complete (11–12 days), lacunae form in the polar syncytiotrophoblast. These lacunae develop a brush border and fuse with maternal capillaries, yielding a blood-filled space which will become the intervillous space. At 13 days, *primary* villous stems are formed with a lining of syncytiotrophoblast and a core of cytotrophoblast and mesoderm. The cytotrophoblast grows as 'columns' through the syncytiotrophoblast to make contact with maternal decidua, and then forms a 'shell' enclosing the lacunae and syncytiotrophoblast (Figs. 1.13, 1.14). The shell is penetrated by maternal spiral arteries and venules. The entire embryo is now buried and the decidua has three regions: the basalis at the deepest embryonic pole, the capsularis over the rest of the chorion, and the parietalis over the remainder of the uterus other than the implantation site (the parietalis fuses with the capsularis in the 5th month and obliterates the uterine cavity). During the early second trimester a second wave of trophoblast invasion takes place from the trophoblast wall.

During the 3rd week of embryonic life the villous stems become vascularised and establish continuity with other vessels developing in the body stalk. The primary villous stems give off syncytial sprouts, which rapidly acquire a cytotrophoblast and then a mesenchymal core to become the *primary villi*. These are true villi as opposed to the primary villous stems, which constitute a supporting framework. After day 21, the villi adjacent to the uterine cavity degenerate to form the chorion laeve; this process is complete by 8–10 weeks. The villi on the decidual side, the chorion frondosum, proliferate to form the placenta. Growth occurs by fresh villus formation from the villous stems and progressive arborisation of previously formed villi. The villous stems

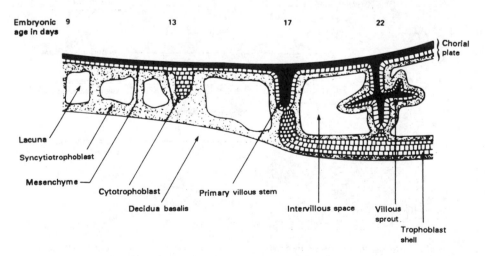

Fig. 1.13. Formation of stem villi and primary placental villi.

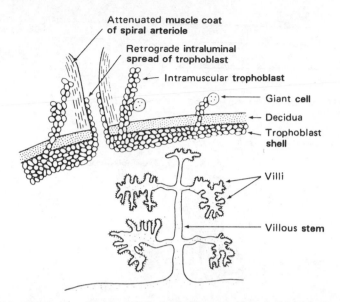

Fig. 1.14. Trophoblast invasion. Cells from the trophoblast shell invade deeply into maternal tissues. Some penetrate the myometrium itself, where they form giant cells. Others invade the lumen of spiral arterioles. As they do so the tunica muscularis of these vessels degenerates (fibrinoid necrosis), producing a loss of resistance in the placental circulation. This process is diminished in many patients who develop pre-eclampsia and asymmetrical growth retardation.

themselves undergo further division. The primary stems break up into a number of secondary stem villi just below the chorial plate. After a short lateral course these give rise to tertiary stems which sweep down through the intervillous space and turn back on themselves near the maternal surface (Fig. 1.15). It is from these tertiary stems that the placental villi arise.

By 12 weeks, the placenta has achieved its definitive form (and thickness, because subsequent growth is circumferential). Initially placental growth is more rapid than that of the fetus, but by 17 weeks they have equal weight. By term, the placenta is one-sixth of the fetal weight.

Multiple pregnancy

Fertilisation of two oocytes leads to the formation of dizygotic (binovular) twins. Monozygotic (identical) twins result from fission of a single embryo, which usually occurs soon after implantation. In Caucasians the incidence of twins at birth is 1 in 80 and a third of these are monozygotic. The incidence of spontaneous triplets (i.e. in the absence of gonadotrophin therapy) is 1 in 8000. In Negroes the incidence of twins is greater, and in Orientals it is lower.

Dizygotic twins have completely separate membranes (amnion and chorion) and amniotic sacs; the two placentas may be contiguous but they are structurally and functionally distinct. The situation in monozygotic twins depends on

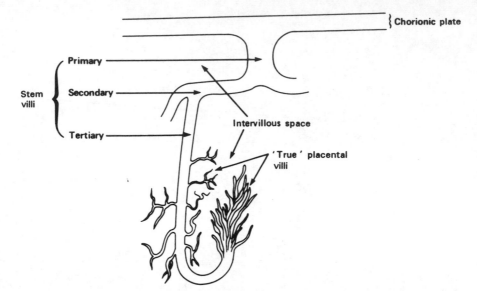

Fig. 1.15. Formation of tertiary stem villi. The stem villi provide the supporting architecture of the placenta.

the stage at which the division of the embryo occurs. Separation at 7–10 days is commonest (two-thirds) and yields a single chorion (monochorionic) and placenta with two amnions (diamnionic) and amniotic cavities. Separation after formation of the amnion is rare and results in both twins in a single amniotic sac (or even incomplete separation with conjoined twins). Separation during the morula stage leads to formation of two placentas and two chorions.

Monozygotic but non-identical twins may occur from an egg fertilised by two sperms. The majority (96%) of hydatidiform moles are 46,XX and result from duplication of a haploid sperm in an empty ovum (diploid androgenesis). XY moles (4%) result from fertilisation of an empty ovum by two spermatozoa (dispermy).

Further development of the embryo

A longitudinal thickening of the posterior part of the embryonic disc develops as the primitive streak (Fig. 1.16). Cells spread out laterally from this to form a layer of mesoderm separating the endoderm and ectoderm (Figs. 1.17–1.19). These three germ layers then give rise to the various organs and tissues. The ectoderm develops into the entire nervous system, epidermis and lens of the eye. The endoderm develops into the lining of the intestinal and respiratory tracts and associated organs (liver, thyroid, pancreas and lungs). The dermis, skeleton, connective tissue, muscle, vascular and urogenital systems arise from mesoderm. The cavity that later divides the somatic and visceral sheets of intra-embryonic mesoderm is the coelom.

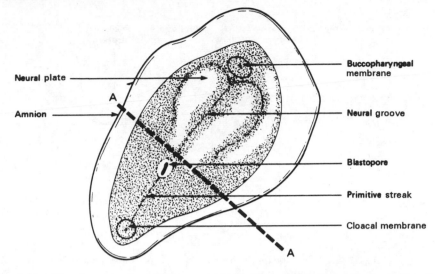

Neural plate

Amnion

A

Buccopharyngeal membrane

Neural groove

Blastopore

Primitive streak

Cloacal membrane

A

Fig. 1.16. Dorsal aspect of an 18-day presomite embryo. AA indicates the level of section in Fig. 1.17.

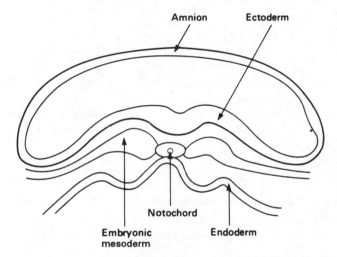

Amnion   Ectoderm

Notochord

Embryonic   Endoderm
mesoderm

Fig. 1.17. Section of the presomite embryo at the level indicated in Fig. 1.16.

The primitive streak becomes prominent during the 3rd week postconception (5th week gestational age). Subsequent events are summarised in Table 1.3.

The placenta

Structure of the mature placenta

The placenta is composed of some 200 *lobules*. Each of these represents the system arising from a primary stem villus. The tertiary stems are arranged in

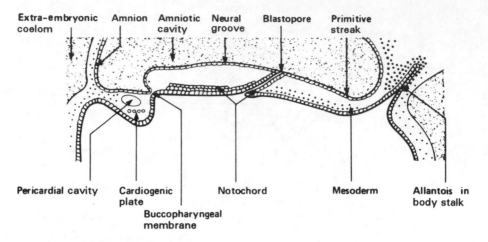

Fig. 1.18. Schematic longitudinal section of a presomite embryo.

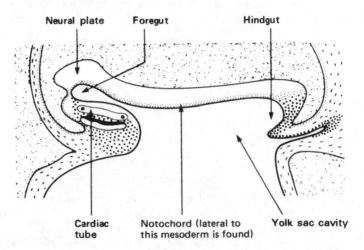

Fig. 1.19. Longitudinal section of a 7-somite embryo; 24 days of embryonic life. Note that the pericardial cavity now lies below the cardiac tube.

circles around a hollow core. There is no relation between lobules or groups of lobules and the *cotyledons* viewed as part of the gross morphology of the placenta.

The two umbilical arteries divide into primary, secondary and tertiary branches corresponding to the stem villi. The tertiary branches break up into a capillary system in the terminal villi. The fetal vessels have no nerve supply beyond the primary stem arteries.

Maternal spiral arterioles terminate via an orifice into the intervillous space and direct a stream of blood towards the chorionic plate. The blood returns through the villus system and is drained by the decidual veins (Fig. 1.20). The wall of the maternal spiral arteries, in both the decidua and the myometrium,

Table 1.3. Principal events of embyonic development

Days 14–21 postconception (see Figs. 1.16-1.18)	Primitive streak becomes prominent in caudal half of disc
	Primitive groove develops in primitive streak as mesoderm forms from primitive streak and moves laterally
	Allantois (diverticulum of endoderm) protrudes into body stalk
	Notochord (precursor of nucleus pulposus) develops from blastopore
	Ectoderm thickens (anterior → posterior) to form neural plate and neural folds
	Mesoderm starts to divide into somites starting at the cephalic end (first four will form occiput)
Days 21–28 postconception (see Fig 1.19)	Neural folds fuse to form neural tube (anterior neuropore closes on days 24–25, and posterior neuropore on days 26–30)
	Heart (mesoderm behind pharynx) is prominent (circulation established)
	Head is very prominent
	Pharyngeal arches form
	Connection between mid-gut and yolk sac constricts
	Otic depression forms
Weeks 4–6 postconception (4–15 mm embryo)	Head proportionately smaller; neck can be recognised
	Optic vesicles appear
	Limb buds appear
	External ear forms
	Formation of face
Weeks 6–8 postconception (15–30 mm embryo)	Digits and eyelids form
	Tail disappears
	All major structures formed. End of embryonic period
	Recognisably human
Weeks 8–12 postconception (30–60 mm)	Ossification centres apparent
	Nails form
	At 9 weeks the paramesonephric (müllerian) ducts reach the urogenital sinus. Thereafter they atrophy in the male and hypertrophy to form the sinovaginal bulbs and later the upper vagina of the female
	External genitalia develop clear-cut features of gender
	Mid-gut withdrawn from umbilical cord

is partially invaded by the cytotrophoblast, leading to a relative dilatation in this site.

Structure of the chorionic villi

The terminal villi are the functional unit of the placenta. Each is surrounded by a continuous outer layer of syncytiotrophoblast and an inner layer of cytotrophoblast; the latter is prominent in the early placenta but is very sparse at term. A basement membrane lies between the trophoblast and the stroma. The stroma contains loose mesenchymal tissue, macrophages (Hofbauer cells) and fetal capillaries (one to six per villus). In the term placenta the syncytial nuclei often form clumps (*syncytial knots*), which protrude from the surface. Some areas of the trophoblast overlying fetal capillaries are very thin (*vasculosyncytial membranes*) and probably specialised for gas transfer. The

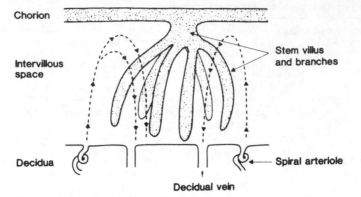

Chorion

Intervillous
space

Stem villus
and branches

Decidua

Spiral arteriole

Decidual vein

Fig. 1.20. Diagram showing maternal circulation through the intervillous (choriodecidual) space.

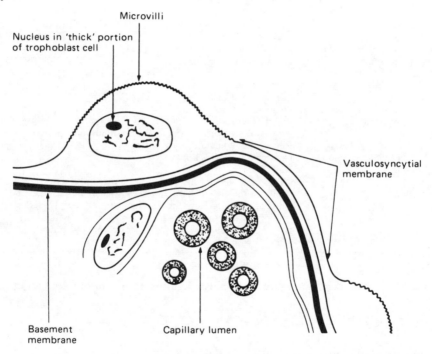

Microvilli

Nucleus in 'thick' portion
of trophoblast cell

Vasculosyncytial
membrane

Basement
membrane

Capillary lumen

Fig. 1.21. Diagrammatic representation of the vasculosyncytial membrane in a portion of a placental villus.

syncytium has a surface of microvilli, but these are absent or sparse over the vasculosyncytial membranes (Fig. 1.21). In the non-membranous areas there is an abundant endoplasmic reticulum, numerous pinocytotic vacuoles and a trans-syncytial canalicular system.

The normal term placenta shows perivillous fibrin deposition, and frequently there is evidence of infarction, intervillous thrombosis and calcification, all of no obvious pathological significance.

Table 1.4.   Products of the placenta

Steroids	Progesterone
	Oestrogens (oestrone, oestradiol, oestriol[a], oestetrol[a])
Protein hormones[b]	Placental lactogen (hPL)
	Chorionic gonadotrophin (hCG)
Enzymes[c]	Heat-stable alkaline phosphatase (HSAP)
	Oxytocinase (cystine aminopeptidase, CAP)
	Histaminase (diamine oxidase, DAO)
Proteins[d]	Pregnancy-specific β_1-glycoprotein (Schwangerschaftsprotein, SP1)
	Pregnancy-associated plasma protein A (PAPP-A)
	Placental protein 5 (PP5)

[a] Dependent on fetal precursors
[b] The placenta also produces peptides which are identical to the ACTH-LPH hormones and to the hypothalamic releasing hormones
[c] The placenta also produces a wide range of 'non-specific' enzymes, especially those related to steroid synthesis (e.g. 3ß-hydroxysteroid dehydrogenase)
[d] A group of proteins identified immunochemically but with no clearly defined biological function. There are at least 12 of these and those listed are the most familiar

Placental synthesis

The syncytiotrophoblast secretes a number of materials, including steroids and a group of proteins which are largely specific to this tissue (Table 1.4). These products are considered to play an important part in adjusting maternal metabolism during pregnancy, though the exact function of individual products is often unclear. In general, the levels of placental steroids are higher in the fetus than in the mother, and the reverse is true for the placental proteins. All products are found in the amniotic fluid at lower levels than in the fetus or the mother.

The main factors controlling the secretion of placental products (and hence maternal levels) are the functional mass of the trophoblast and uteroplacental blood-flow. Maternal levels, therefore, usually correlate with the weight of the placenta and the fetus.

Oestrogens

Oestriol is synthesised in the placenta from fetal precursors: dehydroepiandrosterone (DHA) is produced by the fetal adrenal and hydroxylated in the fetal liver (16OH-DHA); aromatisation of the A-ring of 16OH-DHA in the placenta yields oestriol. Deficiency of fetal adrenal activity (congenital hypoplasia, anencephaly, corticosteroid therapy) is associated with low oestriol levels. In fetal blood, 16OH-DHA circulates as the sulphate conjugate, and the action of a placental sulphatase enzyme is essential to the biosynthetic pathway. In the mother, oestriol is metabolised in the liver, with formation of conjugates (mainly 3-sulphate and 16-glucuronide). These are excreted in urine but a proportion (30%–50%) is excreted in bile and reabsorbed via the enterohepatic circulation.

The other major oestrogens (oestrone, oestradiol) are also secreted by the placenta but have a major contribution from maternal precursors. The minor compound oestetrol is dependent exclusively on fetal precursors. Maternal levels of oestriol (blood and urine) rise progressively throughout pregnancy; the increase continues until term, when oestrogen levels are more than 100 times those in the non-pregnant state.

Progesterone

Progesterone is directly synthesised by the trophoblast. The major excretion product in the mother is pregnanediol. Progesterone levels at term are 10 times the maximal luteal values.

Human placental lactogen (hPL)

Placental lactogen (mol. wt. 21 600; half-life 15 min) has a single chain of 191 amino acids, two disulphide bonds and no carbohydrate residues. It is chemically and functionally similar to pituitary growth hormone and prolactin, but with less biological activity. The levels in maternal blood show a progressive rise, with a plateau after 35 weeks (i.e. a sigmoid curve); only small amounts are excreted in urine. hPL may play a part in the control of carbohydrate and lipid metabolism. In some cases hPL is absent, with no apparent effect on the pregnancy.

Human placental growth hormone (hPGH)

This differs from pituitary GH by 13 amino acids. Its concentration increases progressively in maternal blood during pregnancy, whereas pituitary GH level decreases.

Human chorionic gonadotrophin (hCG)

Chorionic gonadotrophin (mol. wt. 38 400; half-life 5 h (fast component), 24 h (slow component)) consists of two chains of amino acids (α and β), which are linked by non-covalent bonds. Both chains have carbohydrate residues (12% by weight). Chorionic gonadotrophin is chemically and functionally similar to pituitary luteinising hormone. Thus the α-subunit is the common subunit of all the glycoprotein hormones (LH, FSH, TSH, hCG), whereas the β-subunit is similar to that of LH but with an additional 30 amino acids at the carboxy-terminus. Immunoassays directed to the β-subunit are therefore specific for hCG. The levels in maternal blood and urine rise very rapidly in early pregnancy to reach a peak at 12 weeks. hCG may be the luteotrophic signal from the early embryo that prevents the normal degeneration of the corpus luteum. It also has weak thyrotrophic activity.

Placental transfer

Transfer of substances across the placenta depends on the anatomical characteristics of the organ (see above), on the chemical properties of individual substances and on placental perfusion.

Chemical properties affecting placental transfer

1. Lipid solubility facilitates transfer (transfer of many drugs depends on this property).

2. Low molecular weight substances transfer more easily than those of high molecular weight. Water-soluble substances cross readily up to a molecular weight of 100, whereas lipid-soluble substances do so up to a molecular weight of 600 or more. Diffusion is very limited when the molecular weight exceeds 1000.

3. Polar (ionised) substances cross in very small amounts irrespective of their molecular weights (unless specific transport mechanisms exist, as for sodium).

4. Specific transport mechanisms exist for some molecules, which allow them to cross in much larger amounts than their physical properties would otherwise allow (e.g. IgG and purines).

Some small inert molecules, such as water and antipyrine, diffuse readily across the placenta; clearance is limited only by blood-flow (*flow limited*). Other substances do not diffuse rapidly (*permeability limited*) (Fig. 1.22). Some substances which would normally be permeability limited behave in a flow-limited fashion as a result of specific transport mechanisms (e.g. glucose and essential amino acids).

Placental perfusion

The maternal uterine blood-flow reaches 700–750 ml/min at term, of which about three-quarters is directed towards the placenta while the remainder supplies the myometrium. Because the placenta has a low-resistance circulation, high flow rates are recorded even during maternal diastole. Umbilical blood-flow is 350 ml/min. The perfusion pressure across the intervillous space is approximately 70 mmHg (80 mmHg in spiral arteries; 10 mmHg in uterine veins). Like the intervillous space, the umbilical circulation is a low-resistance system.

Placental transfer of individual substances

Water

Water crosses the placenta freely. The exchange of water across the placenta reaches 3.5 l/h by term.

Oxygen and carbon dioxide

Carbon dioxide and oxygen diffuse freely across the placenta and net flow is determined by a pressure gradient. For oxygen the gradient is maintained (a) by the high haemoglobin concentration in the fetus (17 g%), (b) by the greater affinity of fetal haemoglobin (HbF) for oxygen (Fig. 1.23) (the oxygen dissociation curve of HbF is shifted to the left because it is less sensitive to the action of 2,3-diphosphoglyceric acid), and (c) by the Bohr effect (accumulation of carbon dioxide decreases oxygen affinity of maternal haemoglobin and increases the affinity of HbF). However, the partial pressure of oxygen in the fetus is extremely low, about 20 mmHg

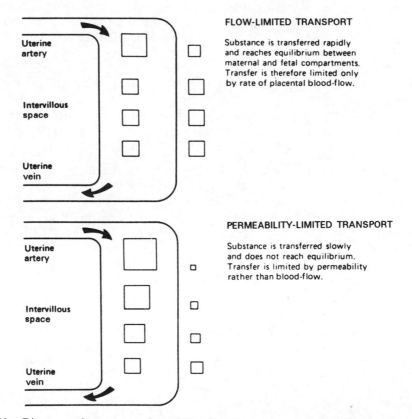

Fig. 1.22. Diagrammatic representation of 'flow-limited' and 'permeability-limited' placental transfer.

(2.7 kPa) in the umbilical arteries and 30 mmHg (4 kPa) in the umbilical vein, whereas uterine venous blood has a P_{O_2} of 40 mmHg (5.3 kPa) (Fig. 1.24). This is the result of shunts, imbalance of perfusion on both sides of the placenta, and oxygen consumption by the placenta itself. Despite the low partial pressure the oxygen *content* of fetal blood is higher than that of the mother (19 ml% as against 16.7 ml%). This is the result of the higher haemoglobin concentration and greater oxygen affinity of fetal blood.

Unlike oxygen, carbon dioxide has similar dissociation curves in fetal and maternal blood. The gradient for carbon dioxide transfer from fetus to mother is increased by the reduced maternal P_{CO_2} of pregnancy, and carbon dioxide diffusion is further facilitated by the increasing carbon dioxide affinity of maternal blood as it releases oxygen (the *Haldane effect*), while the reverse effect occurs in the fetus (the *double Haldane effect*).

Although most of the carbon dioxide in blood is carried as bicarbonate, only the dissolved carbon dioxide can cross the placenta (bicarbonate, being a charged molecule, cannot cross). Equilibrium between carbon dioxide and bicarbonate is established more slowly in the fetus owing to lower concentrations of carbonic anhydrase.

Glucose

The placental transfer of glucose occurs by 'facilitated' diffusion. The polar glucose molecule combines with a carrier protein to form a lipid-soluble complex. The system becomes saturated at a maternal glucose concentration of around 25 mmol/l; below this threshold the gradient across the placenta is small.

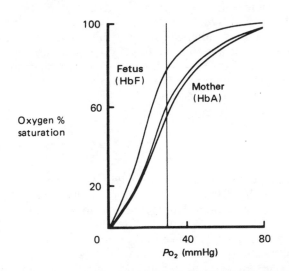

Fig. 1.23. Oxygen dissociation of adult and fetal haemoglobin. HbF constitutes 80% of all circulating haemoglobin in the fetus at term. The greater oxygen affinity of HbF is the result of its lower sensitivity to diphosphoglyceric acid rather than an inherent difference in its oxygen affinity; in free solution the two molecules produce the same oxygen dissociation curves.

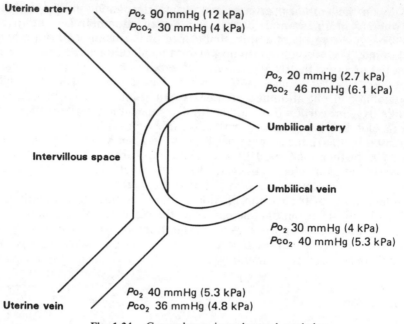

Fig. 1.24. Gas exchange in a placental cotyledon.

Amino acids

Protein turnover in the fetus occurs at ten times the adult rate, and the placenta clears amino acids more avidly than the maternal liver. Acidic non-essential amino acids (e.g. glutamic acid) and neutral straight-chain amino acids (e.g. alanine) are synthesised in the placenta and are not absorbed from maternal serum. The essential neutral branched-chain amino acids (e.g. valine and leucine) and basic amino acids (e.g. lysine and histidine) are transferred to the fetus against a gradient by specific transport mechanisms. As a result the concentration of these 'essential' amino acids is five times higher in the placenta than in maternal blood.

Other nutrients

Free fatty acids cross the placenta freely and levels in the newborn are similar to those in the mother. However, arachidonic acid levels are higher because of synthesis from cholesterol in the placenta. Both fetus and placenta can make fatty acids from glucose.

Water-soluble vitamins are absorbed by active mechanisms, which result in higher concentrations in the fetus. The placenta is impervious to vitamin A, but the fetus synthesises this fat-soluble vitamin from carotene, which crosses the placenta more easily.

Iron and other essential minerals (calcium, iodine) are actively transferred across the placenta.

The permeability of the placenta to drugs is determined by their molecular characteristics. Most drugs will cross to some extent, though some in only very small amounts. For example, neuromuscular blocking agents are highly polarised and therefore cross the placenta in negligible quantities.

The membranes

The amnion

The amnion arises as a layer of epithelial cells between the ectodermal disc of the inner cell mass and the trophoblast (chorion). The amniotic cavity (formed by 7–8 days) lies between the amnion and the ectodermal disc. Proliferation of the mesoderm of the extra-embryonic coelom progressively separates the amnion and chorion.

The amnion has five layers: (a) cuboidal epithelium with a microvillous surface and prominent intracellular canals and numerous vacuoles, (b) basement membrane, (c) a compact layer, (d) a fibroblast layer, and (e) a spongy layer of mucoid reticular tissue (the remnant of the extra-embryonic coelom). There are no blood vessels, lymphatics or nerves.

Table 1.5.   Features of the composition of amniotic fluid

Salts	Sodium and osmolality fall progressively, urea and creatinine increase.
Proteins	Total rises to 26 weeks. Levels around 1/10 that of fetal serum and with a similar pattern. No fibrinogen. α-Fetoprotein levels peak at 10–12 weeks, are much higher than levels in maternal blood but ten-fold less than in fetal blood.
Lipids	Half the lipids are fatty acids and towards term include lecithin (lung surfactant).
Hormones	Similar to those in maternal blood but most are found at lower concentrations. Prolactin levels are 100 times those in the mother or fetus at 25 weeks, but fall to reach similar levels at term. Renin levels are 20 times higher than maternal levels but angiotensin levels are similar. Insulin levels increase throughout pregnancy and are many times higher in the presence of maternal diabetes.
Bilirubin	Decreases progressively in third trimester.
Water	Transfer (exchange) of 250 ml/h with mother and 150ml/h with fetus.
Cells	Cells are more abundant with a female fetus. E cells (epithelial-like): Resistant to trypsin detachment. Poor growth potential. Probably represent unkeratinised fetal epidermal and bladder cells. AF cells (amniotic fluid cells): Grow poorly. Predominant cells in amniotic fluid before culture. Probably amniotic cells. F cells (fibroblast-like): Grow well in culture and are predominantly used for karyotyping. Probably dermal fibroblasts. Glial cells which adhere rapidly to glass are found with neural tube defects.
Antibacterial factors	Zinc-associated β-lysine, lysozyme, peroxidase and interferon-α.

The chorion

The main layer of the chorion is the trophoblast, which arises as a single layer of cells surrounding the blastocyst.

The chorion has four layers: (a) a cellular layer (fibroblasts), (b) a reticular layer, (c) basement membrane, and (d) trophoblast. The trophoblast is a layer two to ten cells thick lying immediately adjacent to the decidua and continuous with the placental trophoblast. No syncytium is apparent, although obliterated chorionic villi may be recognisable. In non-placental areas the term chorion contains no vessels or nerves.

Amniotic fluid (liquor)

In early pregnancy the amniotic fluid is essentially a transudate of fetal serum (via fetal skin and umbilical cord). From the second trimester onwards there are contributions from fetal urine, fetal swallowing (500 ml/day) and excretion of lung fluids. Throughout pregnancy there is a fairly free exchange of materials with the mother (via the membranes).

The volume of amniotic fluid increases progressively (30 ml at 10 weeks; 250 ml at 20 weeks; 750 ml at 30–38 weeks) and then falls slightly at term. Features of the composition of amniotic fluid are summarised in Table 1.5.

Chapter 2

Anatomy

Vulva

The vulva comprises the mons pubis, the labia majora and minora, and the clitoris, and overlaps with the vaginal vestibule.

Labia majora

The labia majora form the lateral boundary of the vulva and extend from the mons pubis to the perineum; their medial aspects consist of stratified squamous epithelium with hair follicles, a thin layer of smooth muscle (tunica dartos), a layer of fascia, adipose tissue and large numbers of sweat and sebaceous glands. They contain numerous nerve endings, some of which are free (pain sensitive) while others are in the form of corpuscles (e.g. Meissner, Merkel, Pacini and Ruffini) (touch and pressure sensitive). The nerve supply is summarised in Table 2.1. The arterial supply comes from the internal and external pudendals and forms a circular rete. The venous drainage forms a plexus with extensive anastomoses to surrounding areas. The lymphatic drainage is summarised in Table 2.2.

Labia minora

The labia minora split into two parts anteriorly, one covering the clitoris and the prepuce and the other forming the central skin covering or frenulum. Posteriorly they meet at the fourchette. They consist of stratified squamous epithelium with sebaceous and sweat glands (lesser vestibular glands), a thin layer of smooth muscle continuous with the tunica dartos, and subcutaneous

Table 2.1. Nerve supply to the vulva

Labia Majora	*Origin*
Anterior hypogastric branch of iliohypogastric	T-12, L-1
Ilio-inguinal	L-1
Genitofemoral (supplying dartos muscle)	L-1, L-2
Sacral plexus:	
Posterior femoral cutaneous nerve	S-1 to S-3
Pudendal nerve	S-1 to S-4
Labia Minora	
As for labia majora, plus perineal branch of pudendal	S-1 to S-4
Clitoris	
Terminal branch of pudendal	S-1 to S-4
Vestibule	
Perineal branch of pudendal	S-1 to S-4

Table 2.2. Lymphatic drainage of the vulva

Area	*Drainage*
Upper 2/3 of labia majora (superficial)	→ symphysis → superficial inguinal nodes
	→ superficial subinguinal nodes
	→ deep subinguinal nodes (Cloquet)
	→ external iliac chain
Lower 1/3 of labia majora (superficial and deep)	(1) → superficial subinguinal nodes → as above
	(2) → posteriorly to rectal lymphatic plexus (inferior haemorrhoidal nodes)
Labia minora	(1) → laterally as labia majora
	(2) → superiorly as lower 1/3 of vagina
	(3) → in midline as upper 2/3 of labia majora
Clitoris	(1) → as upper 2/3 of labia majora
	(2) → some posterior drainage
Vestibule and Bartholin's gland	(1) → anteriorly as labia majora
	(2) → posteriorly to rectal lymphatic plexus

tissue with little or no fat. The epithelium is keratinised on the lateral surface, but changes to mucous membrane on the medial side. The nerve endings are similar to but less abundant than those of the labia majora; the nerve supply is shown in Table 2.1. The arterial supply comes from the arterial rete of the labia majora and from the dorsal artery of the clitoris. The venous plexus drains to the labia majora and to the perineal, vaginal, inferior haemorrhoidal and clitoral veins. Lymphatic drainage is shown in Table 2.2.

Clitoris

The clitoris consists of two small erectile cavernous bodies terminating in a glans consisting of erectile tissue covered by the prepuce. It is attached to the pubic arch by a suspensory ligament and is covered by stratified squamous epithelium with numerous sweat and sebaceous glands except on the glans itself. The nerve endings are similar to those of the labia minora; the nerve supply is shown in Table 2.1. The arterial supply is the dorsal artery of the clitoris (terminal branch of the internal pudendal), which divides into deep and dorsal branches as it enters the clitoris. A venous plexus beginning at the glans drains to the pudendal plexus and thence to the pudendal vein.

Vestibule and Bartholin's gland

The vestibule lies between the labia minora and the hymen (the latter is a perforated membrane which in the parous or postcoital individual consists of skin tags or carunculae myrtiformes). Anteriorly the vestibule includes the urethral orifice, around which open the ducts of the para- and peri-urethral (Skene's) glands. At 5 and 7 o'clock are the duct openings of the larger vestibular (Bartholin's) glands: the latter are arranged as lobules consisting of alveoli lined by cuboidal to columnar epithelium. Their secretion is mucoid and alkaline.

Deep to the vestibule on either side of the commencement of the vagina lies the 'bulb of the vestibule', a flask-shaped mass of erectile tissue covered by the bulbocavernosus muscles, and homologous to the urethral bulb in the male. The skin of the vestibule is stratified squamous epithelium without hair follicles. The nerve endings of the vestibule are mostly free, with few or no corpuscles; the nerve supply is shown in Table 2.1. The arterial supply is in the form of a plexus from the superficial transverse perineal artery, the inferior haemorrhoidal artery, the dorsal artery of the clitoris and the azygous artery of the vagina. The venous drainage is a plexus with extensive anastomoses to the surrounding area. The lymphatic drainage is summarised in Table 2.2.

Vagina

The vagina is 7–10 cm long, the posterior wall being 1.5–2 cm longer than the anterior. The long axis is at an angle of 90° to the cervix. The anterior vaginal wall is in direct relation to the bladder and the urethra throughout its length. The upper quarter of the posterior vaginal wall is related to the peritoneal space (recto-uterine space or pouch of Douglas) and the middle half to the rectum. The lower quarter is separated from the anal canal by the anal sphincters and perineal body. The lateral relations of the vagina are shown in Fig. 2.1.

The vascular supply of the vagina is shown in Table 2.3. The lymphatics form a superficial mucosal and deep muscular plexus on the anterior and posterior surface of the vagina. Drainage is as follows: (a) superior: joins cervical vessels to terminate in medial chain of external iliac nodes; (b) middle: to hypogastric node and nodes in rectovaginal septum; and (c) inferior: as (b) above plus some drainage to the vulva and thence to the inguinal nodes.

Uterus

The uterus is 7.5 cm long and consists of a main part (the body or corpus), a constricted part which also includes the internal os (the isthmus), and a narrow terminal part (the cervix); the portion lying above the openings of the fallopian tubes is known as the fundus. The cervix penetrates the anterior wall but is divided into supravaginal and intravaginal portions. The uterus lies between the bladder and the rectum; it weighs 50 g in nullipara and 70 g in women who have had children. During pregnancy it gains nearly a kilogram in weight

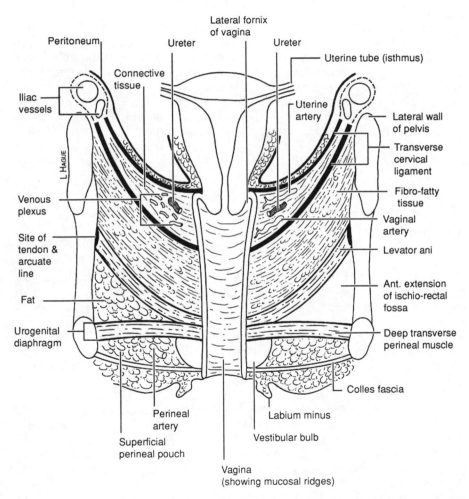

Fig. 2.1. The superolateral and lateral relations of the vagina. Note the transverse cervical ligament with the ureter, uterine artery and vaginal artery. The ligament is dense adjacent to the cervix and lateral fornix of the vagina. It sweeps superolaterally in the shape of a fan to become continuous with the perivascular connective tissue around the iliac vessels.

Table 2.3. Blood supply to the vagina

Arterial
1. Cervicovaginal branch of uterine artery forms coronary artery of cervix (upper part of vagina)
2. Lateral vaginal continuation of inferior vesical arteries (middle part of vagina)
3. Terminal branches of internal iliac arteries (arterio vaginalis) (middle part of vagina)
4. Ascending branches of the middle haemorrhoidal arteries (lower part of vagina)
5. Dorsal artery of the clitoris (lower part of vagina)
6. All of the above form anastomoses with the anterior and posterior azygous arteries of the vagina which lie in the midline

Venous
1. Uterine and cervical veins to hypogastric veins (upper part of vagina)
2. Dorsal vein of clitoris and middle haemorrhoidal veins to internal (lower part of vagina)
3. All these veins originate in extensive plexuses

by hypertrophy and hyperplasia (increase in the size and number of smooth muscle cells).

The external uterine orifice (the external os) is circular in nullipara, but transverse and often fissured in multipara. The intravaginal cervix is usually directed obliquely downwards and backwards, whereas the uterus is usually anteflexed and anteverted (in 20% of women it is retroflexed and retroverted). In most cases the uterus is inclined and rotated slightly to the right because of displacement by the sigmoid colon.

Laterally the uterus is related to the broad ligaments and the uterine arteries which curve upwards in the soft connective tissues of the broad ligaments. The anterior and posterior relations are shown in Fig. 2.2.

The cavity of the uterus is triangular and that of the cervix fusiform. The cervical mucosa in nullipara has a series of 'fern-like' folds (arbor vitae).

The cervix is composed predominantly of fibrous and elastic tissue. The body of the uterus is mostly smooth muscle arranged as an inner longitudinal layer, a layer with multidirectional bundles, and outer layers of circular and longitudinal bundles.

The pregnant uterus

The cervix and isthmus do not change in length during the first trimester of pregnancy. Thereafter the isthmus elongates and its cavity becomes absorbed into the general uterine cavity to form the lower uterine segment. The cervix is 52 mm long until 34 weeks gestation. After 34 weeks the upper part of the cervix is incorporated in the thin segment so that by term the lower segment is made up of 70% isthmus and 30% cervix. Thus in pregnancy the internal os is located in the cervix rather than the isthmus.

Regular contractions called Braxton Hicks' contractions become demonstrable as early as 8 weeks of gestation. They are initiated from pacemakers at the cornua of the uterus and cause progressive attenuation of the lower uterine segment. These are gradually merged into the contractions of labour. Contractions sufficient to raise the intrauterine pressure to 25 mmHg are sufficient to dilate the pregnant cervix. The mean uterine activity during labour is 1100 kPa/15 min and this generates pressures of 60–70 mmHg at the peak of contractions.

During labour the upper segment actively contracts and shortens, while the lower segment passively dilates and lengthens. The progressive shortening of the upper segment is called 'retraction' and is most marked in the third stage of labour. In the latter stage the retraction and high resting 'tone' of the interlacing muscle fibres occlude the intervening vessels, thereby preventing postpartum haemorrhage.

The uterus increases in weight only during the first half of pregnancy; further enlargement in volume is achieved by thinning-out of the uterine walls.

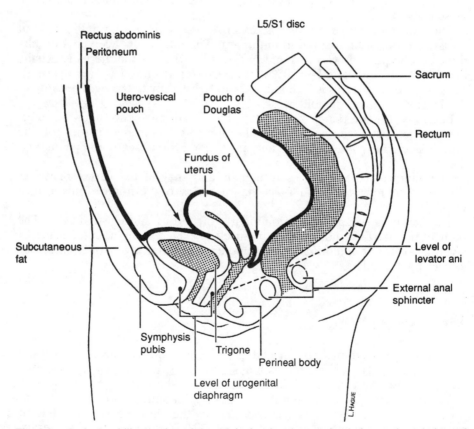

Fig. 2.2. Sagittal, midline section of the pelvis showing the anterior and posterior relations of the uterus. Anteriorly it is related to the bladder, being partly separated by the uterovesical pouch of the peritoneum. Posteriorly it is separated from the rectum by loops of intestine lying in the pouch of Douglas. The peritoneum is reflected onto the posterior fornix of the vagina. It is firmly attached to the fundus of the uterus but loosely arranged in the uterovesical pouch. The levels of the urogenital diaphragm and levator ani are indicated. The septum between the rectum and vagina below the pouch of Douglas is filled with fibro-fatty tissues.

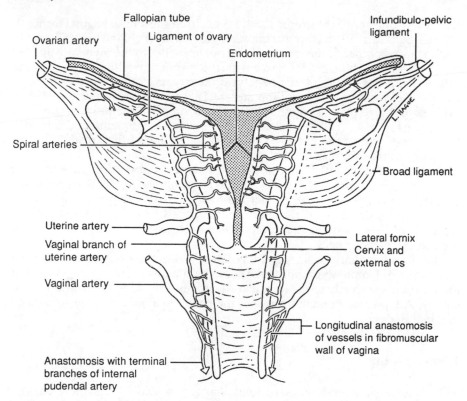

Fig. 2.3. Diagram of the blood supply to the uterus, vagina, ovary and fallopian tubes. The veins follow a similar pattern, terminating in the inferior vena cava. The pattern of the smaller veins is more diffuse and most begin as plexuses (rectal, vesical, etc.). The uterine artery approaches the cervix above the lateral fornix of the vagina and the ovarian artery in the infundibulopelvic ligament. The uterine artery supplies spiral arteries to the endometrium and terminates supplying tubal and ovarian branches. The tubal branch of the ovarian artery anastomoses with the tubal branch of the uterine artery. Note the anastomoses between the uterine artery and the vaginal artery.

Growth of the uterus

The uterus in the newborn is made up of a relatively large cervix and a very small body with no fundus. Subsequently the body grows faster to form two-thirds of the mature organ. At birth the long axis of the uterus corresponds to that of the vagina, but gradually inclines forwards with growth.

Blood supply

The main blood supply (Fig. 2.3) is from the uterine artery, which may arise directly from the internal iliac or arise in common with another branch, especially the superior vesical. The uterine artery runs behind the peritoneum and crosses the transverse cervical ligament. Thereafter, the artery passes anterior to and above the ureter about 1.5 cm from the lateral vaginal fornix. It then ascends in a tortuous course between the two layers of the broad ligament on the lateral border of the uterus, giving out branches to the myometrium and anastomosing at the superior angle with the terminal portion of the ovarian artery. Branches to the uterus penetrate the myometrium and then turn to run parallel with the surface of the uterus. These branches are called arcuate arteries and give off the spiral arteries which supply the endometrium. The uterine artery also gives off branches to the uterine ligaments and a branch to the upper part of the vagina. The 'ovarian' portion of the arcade gives off branches to the fallopian tubes.

During pregnancy the uterine arteries hypertrophy (the luminal area increases by 5 times) and their course is straightened. The vaginal and ovarian arteries do not enlarge, but the ovarian veins are greatly dilated.

The venous drainage of the uterus corresponds to the arterial supply. A network of veins around the cervix communicates with a similar network around the bladder neck.

The main lymphatic drainage of the uterus is into the external and internal iliac group of lymph nodes, although some lymphatics from the upper part of the uterus pass directly to the lateral aortic nodes, following the ovarian blood supply. A few small branches run with the round ligament into the superficial inguinal nodes.

Endometrium

The endometrium undergoes various changes in early pregnancy, characterised principally by proliferation of stromal cells. Under the influence of progesterone these enlarge and store glycogen. The tissue is then referred to as the decidua. The decidual stroma in the first half of pregnancy consists mostly of immune cells. Some of these are T and B lymphocytes, but most are large granular lymphocytes and macrophages. The macrophages are closely associated with the extravillous trophoblast. The large granular lymphocytes are classified as natural killer or activated natural killer cells. It would appear that this cellular immune response is necessary for normal placental development.

The decidua secretes high levels of PP14 (a β-lactoglobulin analogue), insulin-like growth factor binding protein 1 (IGFBP-1), and prolactin.

Fallopian tubes /ovious| uterine nogs
ciuated epithelium

The fallopian tubes lie in the upper margin of the broad ligament and are 10 cm long. The abdominal opening is at the base of a trumpet-shaped expansion with a fimbriated edge, the infundibulum; one of the fimbriae is closely applied to the ovary. From the infundibulum the succeeding parts of the tube are the tortuous ampulla (half of the length), the cord-like isthmus (one-third of the length) and the uterine (intramural) portion (1 cm). The blood supply is from the uterine arteries (medial two-thirds) and the ovarian arteries (lateral one-third). Venous and lymphatic drainage follow a similar pattern.

Ovaries

The ovary is almond shaped (3 cm × 1.5 cm), is attached to the posterior surface of the broad ligament by the mesovarium and occupies the ovarian fossa on the wall of the pelvis (Fig. 2.4). This fossa is bounded anteriorly by the obliterated umbilical artery and posteriorly by the ureter and the internal iliac artery. In early fetal life the ovaries lie in the lumbar region near the kidney.

The surface of the ovary is covered with a layer of cuboidal cells, the germinal epithelium, and beneath this is a thin layer of condensed connective tissue, the tunica albuginea. It has a thick cortex containing follicles and corpora lutea, and a highly vascular medulla. The primordial follicles consist of a central oocyte surrounded by a single layer of flattened follicular cells.

The blood supply is from the ovarian artery and the ovarian vein, which forms from a pampiniform plexus at the hilum. The nerve supply (the ovarian plexus) includes parasympathetic, postganglionic sympathetic and autonomic afferent fibres.

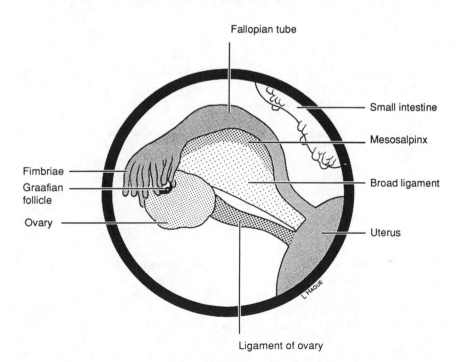

Fig. 2.4. A laparoscopic view of the left ovary and some related structures.

Female urological system

Ureter

The ureter forms as an outgrowth (metanephric diverticulum) from the lower end of the mesonephric duct. The cranial end of the diverticulum gives rise to the pelvis, calices and collecting tubules of the kidney.

Each ureter is 25–30 cm in length. The abdominal part lies on the psoas major, crosses in front of the genitofemoral nerve and is crossed by the ovarian vessels; it enters the pelvis in front of the common or external iliac vessels. The pelvic part follows the anterior border of the greater sciatic notch, turns medially at the ischial spine and runs above the levator ani in the base of the broad ligament (parametrium) to the base of the bladder. In the parametrium the uterine artery lies above and in front of the ureter for 2.5 cm, then crosses the ureter to reach the uterus. The ureter runs above the lateral fornix of the vagina, 2 cm lateral to the cervix, and then turns medially in front of the vagina. It follows an oblique course through the bladder wall.

The ureter has fibrous, muscular and mucosal coats. The muscle has circular and longitudinal layers; only the longitudinal fibres are present in the part traversing the bladder wall. The mucosa consists of transitional epithelium. The blood supply comes from the abdominal aorta and the renal, ovarian, common and internal iliac, vesical and uterine arteries. The nerve supply is both sympathetic and parasympathetic and arises from the renal, aortic, and superior and inferior hypogastric plexuses (T-10 to S-4).

Bladder

The bladder is derived in part from the urogenital sinus and in part from the ends of the mesonephric ducts. It is continuous with the allantoic duct, which persists as a partly canalised fibromuscular band, the urachus, joining the apex of the bladder to the umbilicus.

The bladder wall has three layers: serous, muscular and mucosal. The serous layer is the peritoneal covering of the superior surface. The smooth muscle (detrusor) has internal and external longitudinal layers and a middle circular layer; fibres from the external layer pass with the pubovesical ligaments to the pubic bones. The mucosa is a transitional epithelium which is loosely attached to the muscle except over the trigone (the triangular area bounded by the orifices of the ureters and urethra), where it is firmly attached. There are no true glands although occasional 'mucous follicles' may be found near the urethra.

The blood supply is from the superior and inferior vesical arteries and from small branches from the obturator, inferior gluteal, uterine and vaginal arteries. The veins form a plexus on the inferolateral surface. The parasympathetic nerves (S-2 to S-4, nervi erigentes) convey motor fibres to the detrusor. The sympathetic nerves (T-11, T-12, L-1, L-2) may have the opposite effect, but their main function is vasomotor control. Afferent sensory fibres run with both the sympathetic and the parasympathetic nerves, pain fibres being predominantly in the latter.

Urethra

The female urethra is 4 cm long and is embedded in the anterior wall of the vagina (Fig. 2.5). The smooth muscle layer is continuous with that of the bladder and there is no separate internal sphincter at the junction with the bladder. The urethra is surrounded by two layers of striated voluntary muscle. The intramural layer (the 'external sphincter') consists of slow twitch muscle fibres which exhibit tonic activity at rest. The nerve supply is direct from S-2 to S-4. Together with the bladder neck, this layer is responsible for urethral continence at rest. The peri-urethral striated muscle is supplied by the perineal branch of the pudendal nerve and is responsible for augmenting urethral closure during stress events. Between the muscle and the mucosa is a thin layer of spongy erectile tissue. The mucosa has a transitional epithelium near the bladder neck, grading to a non-keratinised stratified squamous epithelium near the external orifice. On the posterior wall is an epithelial fold, the urethral crest. There are numerous mucosal glands; near the lower end the ducts of these join to form the two para-urethral (Skene's) ducts, which end in an aperture lateral to the external orifice.

The arterial and venous blood supply to the upper third of the urethra is

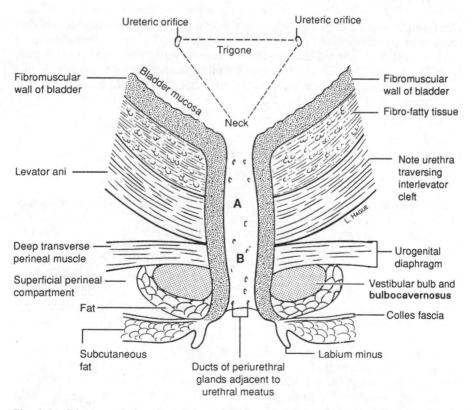

Fig. 2.5. Diagram of the intrapelvic and perineal sections of the urethra traversing the interlevator cleft and the urogenital diaphragm. The wall of the urethra consists of fibromuscular tissues and a cavernous venous plexus.

associated with that of the bladder, and the lower two-thirds with that of the anterior vaginal wall and clitoris. Lymph drainage of the urethra is via the bladder to the external iliac chain. The sensory nerve supply of the urethral mucosa is predominantly from the perineal branch of the pudendal nerve.

Micturition

The normal bladder fills without a rise in intravesicular pressure. This is the result of progressive relaxation of the detrusor smooth muscle, which occurs partly under the influence of the sympathetic nervous system. Sensation of bladder filling does not occur until a volume of 350 ml is reached, and the maximum capacity is 500–600 ml (when acute discomfort occurs). Voluntary voiding is controlled by the pontine micturition centre, which produces contraction of the detrusor muscle and simultaneous urethral relaxation; these continue until the contents of the bladder have been completely expelled, leaving a negligible residual volume.

Continence

Continence of urine depends on urethral pressure being maintained at a higher level than intravesicular pressure. This is achieved by active contraction of both smooth and striated muscles of the urethral wall, with some contribution from the pelvic floor. Thus, when abdominal pressure rises suddenly during coughing, sneezing or straining, urethral pressure also rises to exceed abdominal pressure and prevent urine loss.

Levator ani muscles (pelvic diaphragm)

The levator ani muscles arise from a line beginning on the posterior surface of the superior ramus of the pubis and passing over the internal surface of the obturator foramen (arcus tendineus) to the ischial spine. From this line the fibres sweep inferiorly and posteriorly to interdigitate in the midline and insert into: (a) the pre-anal raphe (perineal body); (b) the wall of the anal canal (deep external sphincter); (c) the ano-coccygeal raphe; and (d) the lower part of the coccyx (Fig. 2.6). The levator muscles have sphincteric action for the vagina. The nerve supply is from the third and fourth sacral nerves. The muscles of the lateral pelvic wall are shown in Fig. 2.7.

The most medial portion of the levator ani is referred to as the pubo-coccygeus and is inserted in front of the rectum. The next portion is the puborectalis, which inserts into the rectum and the first part of the raphe behind the rectum. The most posterior portion is the iliococcygeus, which inserts into the anococcygeal raphe and the coccyx.

The levator ani muscles form the funnel-shaped pelvic diaphragm. Contraction of the abdominal wall, as in straining or coughing, relaxes the

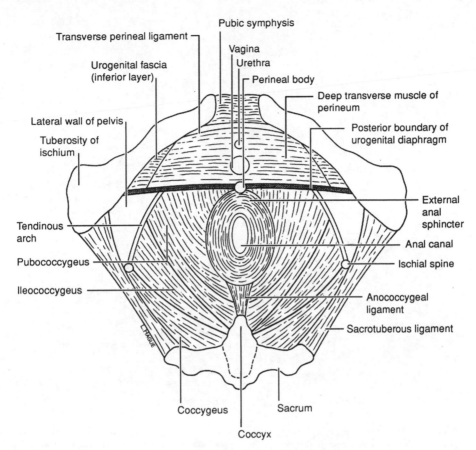

Fig. 2.6. The levator ani muscles viewed from below. The pubococcygeus and ileococcygeus are components of the levator ani, partly arising from the tendinous arch. The cut edge of the urogenital diaphragm can be seen, partly covered by the inferior layer of the urogenital fascia.

levator muscles and thus the angle between the rectum and the anus is diminished.

Perineum

The perineum is bounded by the levatores ani above, by the vulva and anus below, and by the pelvic outlet (subpubic angle, ischiopubic rami, ischial tuberosities, sacrotuberous ligaments and coccyx) laterally. It is divided into a urogenital triangle anteriorly and an anal triangle posteriorly. There is a superficial fascia of fat and a deeper membranous fascia (the fascia of Colles), which extends over the pubis as the fascia of Scarpa.

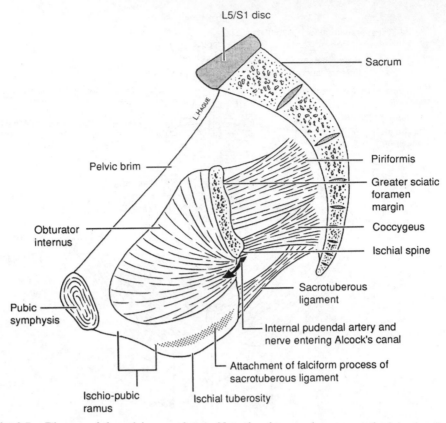

Fig. 2.7. Diagram of the pelvic musculature. Note the obturator internus on the lateral wall of the pelvis with its tendon traversing the lesser sciatic foramen, the piriformis traversing the greater sciatic foramen, and the coccygeus attached to the ischial spine. The internal pudendal artery and nerve traverse the lesser sciatic foramen to lie in Alcock's canal adjacent to the obturator internus. In this position, the obturator internus forms the lateral wall of the ischiorectal fossa.

Urogenital triangle (Fig. 2.8)

The urogenital triangle contains the termination of the vagina and urethra, the crura of the clitoris surrounded by the ischiocavernosus muscles, the bulb of the vestibule surrounded by the bulbocavernosus muscles, Bartholin's glands, the urogenital diaphragm, and the superficial and deep perineal pouches.

Urogenital diaphragm (triangular ligament) (Fig. 2.8)

The urogenital diaphragm is a sheath of muscle enclosed between two triangular fascial membranes. The muscle is formed by the deep transverse perineal muscle and fibres from the sphincter urethrae. The superior layer is the thin fascia bridging the gap between the anterior portions of the levatores ani. The inferior fascial layer is tough and fibrous.

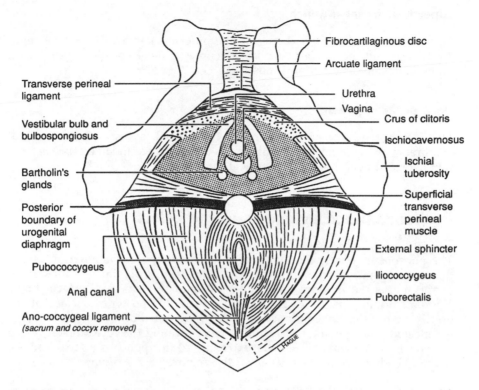

Fig. 2.8. Diagram of the contents of the superficial perineal pouch, part of the pelvic diaphragm, the perineal body and the posterior edge of the urogenital diaphragm. The inferior layer of the diaphragmatic fascia has been removed.

Muscles of the perineum

The *ischiocavernosus muscle* arises from the medial aspect of the inferior ischial ramus and ensheaths the crus clitoridis. It compresses the crus, and by blocking the venous outflow promotes erection of the clitoris.

The *bulbocavernosus muscle* originates in the perineal body, where it interdigitates with the external anal sphincter. It surrounds the bulb of the vestibule and inserts into the body of the clitoris.

The *superficial transverse perineal muscle* radiates from the perineal body to the ischial ramus.

The *deep transverse perineal muscle* has the same origin and insertion but lies deep to the inferior fascia of the urogenital diaphragm.

Perineal body

This is a fibromuscular mass into which the bulbocavernosus, transverse perineal, external anal sphincter and levator ani muscles insert.

Superficial perineal pouch

This is a potential space between the inferior fascia of the urogenital diaphragm and the fascia of Colles. It contains the Bartholin's glands and superficial transverse perineal muscles.

Deep perineal pouch

This is a potential space between the two fascial layers of the urogenital diaphragm and contains the membranous urethra surrounded by the external sphincter and deep transverse perineal muscles.

Peritoneum and ligaments of the pelvis

The peritoneum covers the uterus with the exception of the anterior part of the supravaginal cervix and the intravaginal cervix. From the anterior surface of the uterus the peritoneum is reflected onto the superior surface of the bladder, forming the uterovesical pouch. From the posterior surface of the uterus the peritoneum continues onto the upper third of the vagina before it is reflected onto the anterior rectal surface, forming the rectovaginal pouch (or pouch of Douglas). The lower extremity of this pouch is attached to the perineal body by connective tissue of the rectovaginal septum.

Broad ligament

From the lateral borders of the uterus two layers of peritoneum on each side are reflected to the lateral pelvic walls, forming the broad ligaments. These peritoneal folds include loose connective tissue, referred to as parametrium, which merges inferiorly with extraperitoneal connective tissue. The upper lateral border of the broad ligament forms the infundibulopelvic fold and contains the ovarian vessels in their course from the side wall of the pelvis. The ovary is attached to the posterior layer of the broad ligament by a short double fold of peritoneum (the mesovarium), and the portion of the broad ligament above this is the mesosalpinx. The top of the broad ligament envelops the fallopian tubes. Below and in front of the fallopian tube is the round ligament and below and behind it is the ovarian ligament, all enclosed in the broad ligament.

Vestigial remnants of the mesonephric bodies and ducts (wolffian ducts, duct of Gartner) are contained within the broad ligament. Remnants of the mesonephric body lie above and lateral to the ovary (the epoophoron and hydatid of Morgagni) and between the ovary and uterus (the paroophoron).

Round ligament

The round ligament attaches to the uterine body below and in front of the fallopian tube. It is 12 cm long and passes through the broad ligament to the lateral wall of the pelvis, where it crosses the psoas and external iliac vessels. It hooks round the inferior epigastric arteries to the deep inguinal ring, passes through the inguinal canal and fans out into the labium majus. It is composed mainly of fibrous tissue, with some smooth muscle at the uterine end and some striated muscle at the labial end.

Ligaments formed from pelvic fascia

The connective tissue covering the levator ani is condensed into musculo-fibrous bands in three areas: (a) the transverse cervical ligament (cardinal ligament) arising from the arcuate line on the side wall of the pelvis; (b) the pubocervical ligaments arising from fascia over the pubic bone and passing around the bladder neck; and (c) the uterosacral ligaments (posterior part of the cardinal ligaments) arising from the sacral promontory. All three ligaments insert into the upper vagina and supravaginal cervix.

Blood supply to the female pelvis

The blood supply to the female pelvis is shown in Fig. 2.3. The aorta divides at the level of the fourth lumbar vertebra and the common iliac artery at the level of the lumbosacral intervertebral disc. Continuing vessels leave the pelvis through the obturator foramen (obturator artery), behind the inguinal ligament (femoral artery) and through the greater sciatic foramen (superior and inferior gluteal arteries; internal pudendal artery). The internal pudendal artery curves round the back of the ischial spine and enters the perineum through the lesser sciatic foramen and pudendal canal.

Lymphatic drainage of the female pelvis

The lymphatic drainage of the pelvis begins as plexuses in the individual organs and generally follows the line of the blood vessels. Major and fairly constant groups of nodes include the common iliac, the external iliac (collecting from the inguinal group), the internal iliac, the obturator, and the median and lateral sacral.

Nerve supply to the female pelvis

The nerve supply to the pelvis is broadly arranged as the lumbar and sacral plexuses (Table 2.4) formed from ventral rami of spinal nerves. (Dorsal rami are smaller and supply skin and muscle of posterior aspects of the trunk and buttocks.) The genital branch of the genitofemoral nerve (L-1, L-2) passes through the inguinal canal (accompanying the round ligament)

Table 2.4. Origin and branches of the lumbar and sacral plexuses

Lumbar plexus	
Muscular	T-12, L-1 to L-4
Iliohypogastric	L-1
Ilio-inguinal	L-1
Genitofemoral	L-1, L-2
Lateral cutaneous of thigh	L-2, L-3
Femoral	L-2 to L-4
Obturator	L-2 to L-4
Accessory obturator	L-3, L-4
Sacral plexus	
Muscular	L-4, L-5, S-1, S-2
Superior and inferior gluteal	L-4, L-5, S-1, S-2
Sciatic	l-4, L-5, S-1 to S-3
Perforating cutaneous	S-2, S-3
Pudendal	S-2 to S-4
Levator ani, coccygeus, sphincter ani	S-4
Pelvic splanchnics	S-2 to S-4
Coccygeal plexus	S-4, S-5, coccygeal nerve

to supply the labia majora and mons pubis. The pudendal nerve (S-2 to S-4) leaves the pelvis through the greater sciatic foramen, passes through the lesser sciatic foramen into the pudendal canal, and supplies the skin of the anus and external anal sphincter (inferior rectal nerve), the lower third of the vagina and the labia, the clitoris, the cavernous muscles, the external urethral sphincter and the anterior part of the levator ani.

The parasympathetic nerve supply to the pelvis emerges as myelinated, preganglionic nerves (efferent) with the ventral rami of S-2 to S-4 to constitute the pelvic splanchnic nerves. The ganglia are situated in the walls of the organs supplied (motor or inhibitory fibres to the rectum, bladder and erectile tissue of the clitoris; vasodilator fibres to the ovary and uterus).

The sympathetic nerve supply to the pelvis arises from the sympathetic nerve trunks, which have four ganglia in the lumbar region and four or five in the sacral region. The origin of the pelvic sympathetic fibres is from T-11 to L-2. From the ganglia, grey rami communicantes pass to the lumbar and sacral spinal nerves while other fibres form the hypogastric plexus. The upper part of the latter is sometimes referred to as the presacral nerve, and divides inferiorly to give the left and right hypogastric nerves (plexuses) lying on the side of the rectum, cervix and vagina. In turn, these give rise to plexuses related to each organ (the middle rectal, vesical, uterovaginal), from which nerves pass with arteries to the respective organ. The ganglia of the sympathetic nerves lie either in the main paravertebral nerve trunks or in the subsidiary plexuses: thus all fibres are non-myelinated and postganglionic when they reach their target organs. The sympathetic nerves provide vasomotor control (vasoconstriction), together with control of the smooth muscle of the uterus and bladder.

Afferent autonomic fibres travel in both the hypogastric plexus (sympathetic) and the pelvic splanchnic nerves (parasympathetic) to reach cell bodies in the spinal and cranial ganglia. These fibres are concerned with visceral sensation (e.g. bladder and rectal distension, sexual excitement, cervical stretching, uterine contractions).

Some general features of the autonomic nervous system are summarised in Table 2.5.

Table 2.5. Some general features of the autonomic nervous system. Note that each preganglionic neuron may synapse with 15–20 postganglionic neurons

Sympathetic	Parasympathetic
Preganglionic fibres from lateral horn of spinal column emerge with T-1 to L-2	Preganglionic fibres with cranial nerves and S-2 to S-4
Preganglionic fibres enter sympathetic trunks via white rami and synapse in the trunk or in more peripheral ganglia (e.g. coeliac and hypogastric (i.e. at a distance from organ innervated)	Ganglia situated immediately adjacent to or in the wall of the organ supplied
Preganglionic nerve terminal releases acetylcholine (nicotinic receptor): postganglionic releases noradrenaline (except supply to sweat glands, which is cholinergic)	Preganglionic and postganglionic terminals release acetylcholine (ganglionic receptor is nicotinic)
Peripheral receptors are: α (vasoconstrictor, iris dilatation, bladder sphincter contraction), β_1 (increased heart rate, lipolysis) or β_2 (vasodilatation, bronchodilatation, uterine relaxation, glycogenolysis)	Peripheral receptors are muscarinic (visceral; blocked by atropine) or nicotinic (neuromuscular junctions)

Pelvic skeleton

The bony pelvis is made up by the innominate bone, the sacrum and the fifth lumbar vertebra.

The *innominate bone* consists of:

1. *Ilium*. The most prominent feature is the iliac crest: projections at each end of this are the anterior and posterior superior iliac spines. The medial surface presents the iliac fossa, the iliac tuberosity and the auricular surface, which articulates with the sacrum.

2. *Ischium*. This consists of a body and a ramus: the body forms part of the acetabulum, and the ramus fuses with the ramus of the pubis to complete the obturator foramen. The most prominent features are the ischial spine and the ischial tuberosity.

3. *Pubis*. This consists of a body and two rami. The superior ramus joins the ilium and ischium to form the acetabulum; the inferior ramus joins the ramus of the ischium to complete the obturator foramen. The upper border of the body forms the pubic crest and pubic tubercle, and the medial surface forms a cartilaginous joint with the opposite pubis (the pubic symphysis).

These are joined by bone in the adult and cartilage in the young; the junction is in the acetabulum and all three parts contribute to this (Figs. 2.9 and 2.10).

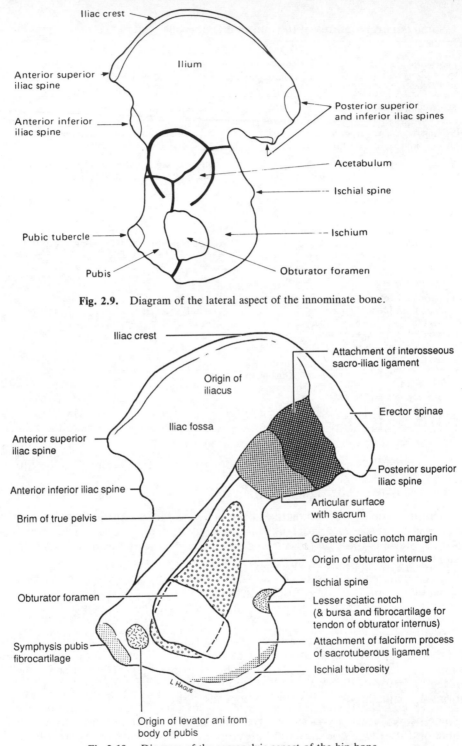

Fig. 2.9. Diagram of the lateral aspect of the innominate bone.

Fig 2.10. Diagram of the sacropelvic aspect of the hip bone.

Table 2.6. Principal structures attached to the pelvic bones

Ilium	
Iliac crest	Quadratus lumborum, transversus abdominis, latissimus dorsi, obliquus externus and internus
Lateral surface (gluteal)	Gluteal muscles
Pelvic surface (iliac fossa)	Iliacus
Iliac tuberosity	Erector spinae, sacro-iliac and iliolumbar ligaments
Anterior inferior iliac spine	Rectus femoris
Anterior superior iliac spine	Inguinal ligament, sartorius
Ischium	
Ischial spine	Coccygeus, levator ani, sacrospinous ligament
Ischial tuberosity	Semimembranosus, semitendinosus, biceps femoris, sacrotuberous ligament
Body	Quadratus femoris, ischiofemoral ligament
Ramus	Adductor magnus, obturator externus and internus, gracilis, ischiocavernosus, transverse perineals, fascia lata of thigh
Pubis	
Pubic tubercle	Inguinal ligament
Pubic crest	Rectus abdominis, pyramidalis
Inferior ramus	Gracilis, adductor brevis, obturator internus and externus
Sacrum	
Pelvic surface	Piriformis, coccygeus
Posterior surface	Erector spinae, multifidus, gluteus maximus, sacro-iliac ligament

The *sacrum* consists of the five sacral vertebrae joined by bone in the adult and cartilage in the young. There are four sacral foramina communicating with the sacral canal. The upper border of the pelvic surface is the sacral promontory. The sacrum articulates above with the fifth lumbar vertebra, laterally with the ilium and below with the coccyx (three to five fused coccygeal vertebrae).

The structures attached to the pelvic bones are listed in Table 2.6.

Foramina and canals in the pelvis

Obturator foramen. This is bordered by the ischium and pubis and is occupied by a fibrous sheet, the obturator membrane. Superiorly there is a small gap (canal) which communicates between the pelvis and the thigh and carries the obturator artery, vein and nerve.

Greater sciatic foramen. This is formed by the greater sciatic notch (ilium and ischium), the sacrotuberous and sacrospinous ligaments, and the ischial spine (Fig. 2.11). It transmits the piriformis muscle, the superior and inferior gluteal vessels and nerve, the internal pudendal vessels and nerve, the sciatic and posterior femoral cutaneous nerves, and the nerves to the quadratus femoris.

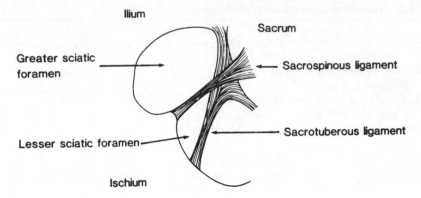

Fig. 2.11.   The greater and lesser sciatic foramina.

Lesser sciatic foramen.   This is bounded by the ischium and ischial spine (Fig. 2.11) and by the sacrotuberous and sacrospinous ligaments. It transmits the tendon of the obturator internus, and the internal pudendal vessels and nerve. The nerve to the obturator internus passes lateral to the internal pudendal vessels and nerves, and innervates the obturator internus on the wall of the ischiorectal fossa.

Pudendal canal.   This is a sheath of fascia on the lateral wall of the ischiorectal fossa, transmitting the internal pudendal vessels and nerve.

Sacral foramina.   There are four pairs of these on each of the dorsal and ventral surfaces of the sacrum. They communicate with the sacral canal through the intervertebral foramina and transmit the dorsal and ventral rami of the first four sacral spinal nerves.

Sacral canal.   The sacral canal is formed by the vertebral foramina of the sacral vertebrae; the lower opening is the sacral hiatus. As the spinal cord ends at the first lumbar vertebra, the sacral canal contains only nerve roots (cauda equina) and the filum terminale. The subarachnoid space extends to the lower border of the second sacral vertebra, and below this the dura mater and arachnoid form a closely applied covering of the filum terminale as it descends to its attachment on the first coccygeal segment.

General features of the bony pelvis

The true (or lesser) pelvis consists of a cavity with upper and lower openings; typical measurements are shown in Table 2.7. The *superior pelvic aperture* (pelvic inlet, pelvic brim) is bounded by the sacral promontory, the arcuate line of the ilium, the iliopectineal line and the rest of the pubis. The *cavity* is short and curved. Anteriorly it is bounded by the body of the pubis and its rami and symphysis, posteriorly by the sacrum and coccyx, and laterally by the fused ilium and ischium. The *inferior pelvic aperture* (pelvic outlet) is bounded by three wide notches: the pubic arch and the two sciatic notches. For practical

Table 2.7. Dimensions of the female pelvis

Site	Centimetres
Pelvic inlet	
Anteroposterior (true conjugate) (sacral promontory to upper border of pubic symphysis)	11.2
Transverse	13.1
Oblique (iliopubic eminence to opposite sacro-iliac joint)	12.4
Pelvic cavity	
Anteroposterior (3rd sacral segment to posterior surface of pubic symphysis)	13.0
Transverse	12.5
Oblique (lowest point of sacro-iliac joint to midpoint of obturator membrane)	13.1
Pelvic outlet	
Anteroposterior (apex of coccyx to midpoint of lower border of pubic symphysis)	12.5
Transverse (between lower borders of ischial tuberosities)	11.8
Oblique (midpoint of sacrotuberous ligament to junction of opposite ischial and pubic rami)	11.8
Others	
Diagonal conjugate (between sacral promontory and lower border of pubic symphysis)	12.6
Interspinous (between ischial spines)	10.8

Table 2.8. Sex differences

Female	Male
Iliac blades more vertical	Iliac crests rugged
Iliac fossa shallower	
Sacrum broader and less curved	
Sub-pubic arch 80–85°	Sub-pubic arch 50–60°
Ischiopubic rami narrower	
Obturator foramen triangular	Obturator foramen ovoid
	Ischial spines closer
Greater sciatic notch wider	
Greater anteroposterior diameters, especially at lower ends	Cavity longer and more conical

purposes it can be regarded as diamond shaped, the anterior limbs being the ischiopubic rami, and the posterior limbs being the sacrotuberous ligaments with the coccyx in the midline.

Sex differences in the pelvis are listed in Table 2.8.

Fetal skull

The fetal skull consists of the two frontal bones, the two parietal bones and the occipital bone: these are separated by sutures and membranous fontanelles (Fig. 2.12). Certain regions of the skull are designated as the presenting

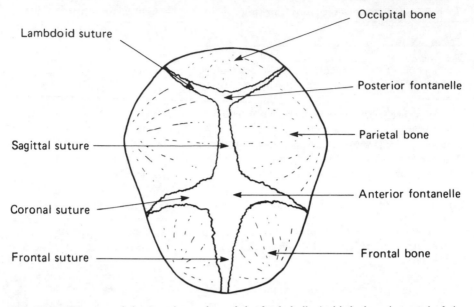

Fig. 2.12. Diagram of the superior surface of the fetal skull. At birth there is a total of six fontanelles.

part during labour: (a) the occiput: the area behind the posterior fontanelle; (b) the vertex: between the anterior and posterior fontanelles and the two parietal eminences; (c) the bregma: the area of the anterior fontanelle; and (d) the sinciput: the area lying in front of the anterior fontanelle, further divided into the brow and face (above and below the root of the nose). The presenting diameter of the fetal skull varies with the presenting part: (a) occipital: suboccipitobregmatic diameter (9.5 cm); (b) vertex: occipitofrontal diameter (11.5 cm); (c) brow: mentovertical diameter (13.0 cm); and (d) face: submentobregmatic diameter (9.5 cm). Two other important diameters are the biparietal (9.5 cm) and the bitemporal (8.0 cm). Moulding during labour may reduce skull diameters by 1–1.5 cm. The parietal bones can readily slide under each other, and the occipital and frontal bones can slide under the parietals.

Microstructure and function of the non-pregnant reproductive tract

Mucosa of the fallopian tubes

The fallopian tubes are lined by a single layer of columnar epithelium with three types of cell: ciliated, secretory and resting ('peg'). The secretory cells are found throughout the tube but are most numerous at the isthmic end; they develop microvilli and become secretory at mid-cycle. Cilia beat asynchronously at about 7 beats/s.

Fallopian tube secretions contain pyruvate, which is an important substrate for the embryo. They contain less glucose, protein and potassium than serum.

Muscular activity of the fallopian tubes

Muscular activity in the infundibulum draws the fimbriae close to the ovary at the time of ovulation. The tube displays both high-frequency/low-amplitude and low-frequency/high-amplitude contractions. The former are more characteristic of the ampulla; the latter occur in the isthmus and may propagate in either direction.

Ovum transport is rapid in the ampulla but a physiological sphincter at the isthmus delays passage into the uterus for 3 days. This area also contains numerous α- (excitatory) and β- (inhibitory) adrenergic receptors. The former are stimulated by the high levels of oestrogen around the time of ovulation.

Endometrium

The endometrium is composed of a basal layer and a stroma covered by columnar epithelium. The latter forms uterine glands, which extend through the stroma into the basal layer. The columnar epithelium includes ciliated cells, which are most numerous near the opening of the glands, and secretory cells with microvilli, which are fully developed during the secretory phase. Some microvilli enlarge at days 20–22 of the menstrual cycle and withdraw fluid from the uterine lumen into large pinocytotic vesicles. Regeneration of the epithelium after menstruation takes place from the epithelium at the base of the endometrial glands.

Following menstruation the epithelium proliferates and the endometrium reaches a thickness of 5 mm. Towards mid-cycle the arterioles take on a spiral form and subnuclear aggregates of glycogen appear in the epithelium. Immediately after ovulation, the fall in oestrogen levels causes a loss of fluid from the endometrium. This shrinkage produces the 'ring sign' on ultrasound. During the luteal phase there is further thickening of the endometrium (10 mm or more) caused by vascular proliferation, oedema of the stroma and accumulation of secretion in the uterine glands. The glands become tortuous, and vacuoles of glycogen push the nuclei to the luminal surface. After day 20 these vacuoles move to the surface and are discharged. Predecidual changes occur in the stroma: the stellate cells become rounder and accumulate lysosomes. The maximum thickness increases with age up to the menopause.

In the final stage of the cycle the coiled arterioles constrict and the superficial zone becomes avascular. There is a loss of interstitial fluid, leucocytic infiltration of the stroma and extravasation of blood as the superficial layers become necrotic. The blood enters the lumen but does not clot. The underlying basal layer remains intact, as do the bases of the glands. Levels of $PGF_{2\alpha}$ in the endometrium rise in the luteal phase and exceed PGE_2 by $25:1$ at the time of menstruation. The former constricts spiral arterioles; the latter relaxes them.

Activity of the myometrium during the reproductive cycle

As in the fallopian tube, high-frequency/low-amplitude and low-frequency propagated contractions occur. The latter originate near the uterotubal junctions and are most prominent during menstruation, when intrauterine pressures similar to or higher than those in labour (about 70 mmHg) are produced. α-Adrenergic receptors stimulate contraction; β-adrenergic receptors have the opposite effect. The uterus, in common with the bronchus but unlike the heart, contains mainly β_2-receptors. Contraction of the uterus is potentiated by $PGF_{2\alpha}$ and, in the non-pregnant state, inhibited by PGE_2. Oxytocin stimulates release of large amounts of $PGF_{2\alpha}$ from the endometrium.

Cervix

The cervix is lined by secretory columnar epithelium arranged as branched glands. This epithelium undergoes only minor changes during the menstrual cycle. The cervical mucus becomes profuse and clear under the action of oestrogen before ovulation. It produces a ferning pattern on drying, exhibits *spinnbarkeit* (by day 14 a single thread may be drawn out to 8 cm) and has an alkaline pH. Once progesterone secretion begins, the cervical mucus becomes thick, opaque, highly cellular and less abundant.

Towards mid-cycle the cervical fluid becomes more hydrated. The macro-molecules (glycoprotein) condense into 'micelles' which are penetrated by a network of channels. These enlarge from 6 μm before ovulation and provide a route for sperm penetration.

Vagina

The wall of the vagina consists of three layers: a mucous membrane, a muscular coat (circular and longitudinal) and a thin connective tissue covering. Striated fibres of the bulbocavernosus and levator ani muscles form sphincters. The striated squamous epithelium has three layers: a basal layer of cuboidal cells, an intermediate layer which is rich in glycogen, and a superficial zone of flat cornified cells with small nuclei. The underlying lamina propria contains collagen and elastic fibres and a rich nerve and blood supply. The superficial zone is best developed at mid-cycle, as reflected by a high karyopyknotic index. This is much lower during the luteal phase, when the vaginal smear contains many more leucocytes. During reproductive life the columnar epithelium of the cervix may encroach upon the vaginal surface of the cervix.

The vagina is normally acid (pH 3.8–4.2) owing to conversion of glycogen to lactic acid in desquamated cells by Döderlein's lactobacillus. Glycogen levels are highest at the time of ovulation. The total number of organisms in vaginal fluid is 10^8–10^9 per ml. The pH rises to 6.5–7.5 during menstruation and after the menopause. Because of the buffering power of seminal plasma, the vagina remains alkaline for 6–8 h after coitus. Vaginal fluid has a higher potassium and lower sodium concentration than plasma. Volatile fatty acids in the vaginal secretions may act as pheromones, stimulating sexual activity. The associated apocrine glands of the vulva secrete undecylenic acid, a fungicidal substance.

Embryology of the genital system

Ovary

Primitive germ cells are first apparent in the endoderm of the yolk sac, from which they migrate to the gut and through the mesentery to the genital ridge on the medial aspect of the mesonephros. The primitive gonad consists of the thickened coelomic epithelium of the genital ridge, the underlying mesoderm and the germ cells, which are now rapidly dividing oogonia. By 5–6 weeks postconception the epithelium has grown inwards as a series of gonadal cords. Further development of these cords (as secondary cords) obliterates the mesenchymal elements. The epithelial elements and oogonia proliferate vigorously up to 14 weeks; the predominance of cortical tissue distinguishes the early ovary from the testis. From this stage stroma cells develop from the mesenchyme in the hilum and spread peripherally. When the process is complete the primary oocytes are surrounded by a ring of epithelial cells (granulosa) embedded in the stroma. The identity of the gonad is apparent by 7 weeks in the testis and 9–10 weeks in the ovary.

At 11–12 weeks the germ cells enter the leptotene stage of the prophase of the first meiotic division. They remain in prophase until ovulation occurs, which may be decades later. The number of germ cells reaches a maximum (7 million in each ovary) at 15–20 weeks, falling to 2 million at birth and 400 000 by puberty. In 45,X Turner's syndrome the oocytes disappear at an accelerated rate and are gone by the age of two.

The early ovary is attached to the inguinal fold and uterus by a fibromuscular gubernaculum along which it descends to its definitive site. The cranial part of the gubernaculum becomes the ovarian ligament and the caudal part becomes the round ligament. The lower end of the gubernaculum is associated with a peritoneal projection, the processus vaginalis, which may persist in the labia majora as the canal of Nuck.

Uterus and fallopian tubes

The paramesonephric (müllerian) duct develops on the lateral aspect of the mesonephros at 5–6 weeks embryonic age and extends caudally to reach the urogenital sinus at 9 weeks (müllerian tubercle). The wolffian duct develops before the paramesonephric ducts and gives out a pouch (the ureteric diverticulum) before entering the urogenital sinus. Subsequently the wolffian system is taken up into the wall of the urogenital sinus and the ureteric opening becomes separated from the wolffian unit. The wolffian system therefore contributes to the ureter, the trigone of the bladder, and in the male the urethra above the level of the ejaculatory duct. At 8 weeks both the müllerian and the wolffian ducts are present and sex differentiation begins. In the female the wolffian ducts degenerate due to a lack of testosterone;

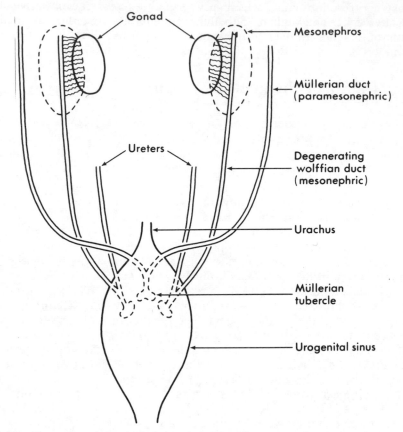

Fig. 2.13. Formation of the müllerian and wolffian duct systems and their entrance into the urogenital sinus. The lower ends of the ureters develop in a diverticulum of the wolffian ducts.

in the male a local effect of testosterone maintains these ducts. The lower portions of the müllerian ducts fuse to form the uterus and cervix while the upper portions remain separate as the fallopian tubes. In the male the müllerian system degenerates under the influence of a glycoprotein inhibitory factor from the Sertoli cells of the testis; this 'müllerian inhibiting factor' is locally active. Remnants of the wolffian duct system may be evident as cysts in the vagina (Gartner's duct); remnants of the wolffian duct and mesonephric tubules may persist in the broad ligament (parovarian cysts).

Various aspects of the development of the genitourinary system are shown diagrammatically in Figs. 2.13–2.15.

Vagina

Paired sinovaginal bulbs on the posterior aspect of the urogenital sinus fuse with the lower end of the müllerian ducts to form the vaginal plate. This consists of solid epithelium, which grows rapidly and then becomes canalised at 16–18 weeks. The vaginal epithelium is greatly hypertrophied in the later months of fetal life. In the mature vagina the upper four-fifths is derived from the müllerian duct and the lower fifth from the urogenital sinus.

External genitalia

The primitive cloaca becomes divided by a transverse septum which fuses with the cloacal membrane (7 weeks). The anterior part is the urogenital sinus and on the external surface is a conical projection, the genital tubercle. Proliferation of the mesoderm leads to formation of the genital folds medially and the genital swellings laterally. At this point (10 weeks) male and female development is identical.

The urogenital sinus has three portions: the upper portion, which will form

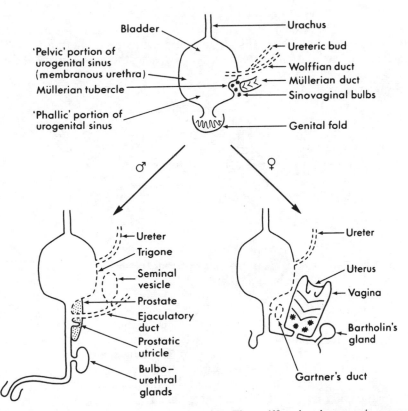

Fig. 2.14. Development of the bladder and vagina. The wolffian duct becomes incorporated into the wall of the urogenital sinus; in this way the ureter and wolffian duct enter the urogenital sinus separately. The area between the two becomes the trigone of the bladder. The upper part of the urogenital sinus forms the remainder of the bladder. The middle portion forms the membranous urethra while the lower portion forms the vestibule in the female and the lower part of the penile urethra in the male. The remainder of the penile urethra is formed from the genital folds. These form the labia minora in the female.

the bladder; the pelvic portion, which will contribute to the urethra and form the prostate gland in the male; and the lower or phallic portion, which will become increasingly shallow to form the vestibule in the female and contribute to the penile urethra in the male. In the female the genital tubercle becomes the clitoris, the genital folds become the labia minora, and the genital swellings become the labia majora. A comparison with developments in the male is shown in Table 2.9.

Normal female development does not depend on gonadal hormones: instead, it is a 'neuter' state which occurs in the absence of the testis. The testis has three endocrine effects: (a) secretion of müllerian inhibiting factor; (b) secretion of testosterone, which directly promotes wolffian developments; and (c) secretion of testosterone, which is converted to dihydrotestosterone by 5α-reductase in the external genitalia and promotes male development at this site.

Anterior abdominal wall

The anterior abdominal wall includes skin, superficial fascia, a muscle/aponeurosis layer, transversalis fascia and peritoneum. There are four main muscles: the internal and external obliques, and the transversus and rectus

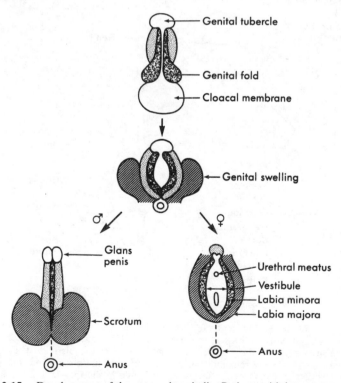

Fig. 2.15. Development of the external genitalia. Patients with intersex states will have a form of development intermediate between the male and the female.

Table 2.9. The differentiation of primitive structures into the male and female gonads and genitalia

Primitive structure	Female	Male
Gonad	Ovary	Testis
Müllerian system (paramesonephric)	Uterus, tubes, upper 4/5 of vagina	Appendix testis, prostatic utricle
Wolffian system (mesonephric)	Occasional remnants (paroophoron, epoophoron), part of bladder and urethra	Epididymis, vas deferens, trigone of bladder and prostatic urethra above the ejaculatory duct
Genital tubercle	Clitoris	Penis
Genital folds	Labia minora	Penile urethra
Genital swellings	Labia majora Bartholin's glands	Scrotum Bulbo-urethral glands

abdominis. All of these are supplied by T-6 to T-2 and L-1. A diagrammatic section through the anterior abdominal wall is shown in Fig. 2.16.

Muscles of the anterior abdominal wall

The *external oblique* (obliquus externus) arises from the lower eight ribs. Some muscle fibres terminate on the iliac crest; the remainder form an aponeurosis which ends medially in the linea alba (a tendinous structure extending from the xiphoid process to the pubic symphysis) and below on the pubic symphysis and pubic crest. Between the pubic tubercle and the anterior superior iliac spine the thickened margin of the aponeurosis forms the inguinal ligament. Just above the pubic crest is a triangular aperture, the superficial inguinal ring; the deep inguinal ring in the transversalis fascia lies above and lateral to this. The inguinal canal runs between these two rings and contains the round ligament (spermatic cord in the male) and the ilioinguinal nerve.

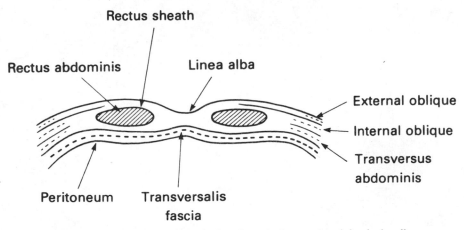

Fig. 2.16. A diagrammatic section through the anterior abdominal wall.

The *internal oblique* (obliquus internus) arises from the lateral two-thirds of the inguinal ligament, from the iliac crest and from the thoracolumbar fascia. It inserts to the lower three to four ribs. Some fibres from the inguinal ligament arch around the round ligament of the uterus and join the aponeurosis of the transversus abdominis to form the conjoint tendon inserting into the pubis.

The *transversus abdominis* arises from the lateral third of the inguinal ligament, the iliac crest, the thoracolumbar fascia and the internal aspects of the lower six costal cartilages. It forms an aponeurosis, the lower fibres of which contribute to the conjoint tendon while the remainder blends with the linea alba in the midline.

The *rectus abdominis* arises by tendons from the pubis and is attached to the fifth to seventh costal cartilages. It has three tendinous intersections and is enclosed by the fibrous rectus sheath. Inside this sheath, behind the rectus muscle, are the superior and inferior epigastric vessels and the terminal parts of the intercostal nerves. The posterior wall of the sheath ends as the arcuate line midway between the umbilicus and the pubic symphysis.

The *pyramidalis* is a triangular muscle in front of the lower part of the rectus abdominis.

Chapter 3
General Physiology and Biochemistry

Cardiovascular system

Heart

During pregnancy the heart is pushed upwards and rotated forwards, with lateral displacement of the left border. The apex beat appears in the fourth rather than the fifth intercostal space. The volume increases by 70–80 ml (12%). All heart sounds are louder and the first sound is split. A systolic ejection murmur is normal, and a diastolic murmur is heard occasionally. The wall on the left ventricle thickens.

The ECG may show low-voltage QRS complexes, deep Q waves, flattening or inversion of the T wave, and depression of the S–T segment. Atrial or ventricular extrasystoles are common.

Cardiac output rises from 7 litres/min at 8–11 weeks to 9 litres/min at 36–39 weeks. The rise is caused by an increased stroke volume (64–71 ml) and an increase in rate (8 beats/min by 8 weeks; 16 beats/min by term). Myocardial contractility is increased. The arteriovenous oxygen difference is reduced in early pregnancy (33 ml/litre) but returns to non-pregnant values at term (45 ml/litre).

Blood pressure

Systolic blood pressure does not change in pregnancy; diastolic pressure is reduced in the first two trimesters and returns to the non-pregnant level at term. The combination of increased cardiac output and decreased diastolic blood pressure indicates that peripheral resistance is reduced. This is caused by the placenta acting as an arteriovenous shunt, together with peripheral vasodilating factors such as oestrogen and progesterone, and increased endothelial synthesis of prostaglandin E_2 and prostacyclins. Blood pressure is lower when the woman is lying down (supine or on her side) than when she is sitting. Both blood pressure and cardiac output are reduced during epidural analgesia.

Venous pressure is increased in the legs during pregnancy, but not in the arms. The increase is due to mechanical obstruction by the uterus and its contents and to the high pressure of venous outflow from the uterus. The rise in venous pressure, together with the fall of colloid osmotic pressure in the blood, explain the leg oedema which occurs in 40% of pregnant women.

Blood-flow in individual organs

Uterine blood-flow increases during pregnancy, reaching values around 700 ml/min at term. Blood-flow also increases in other organs, the largest changes being in the kidneys (up to 400 ml/min) and the skin (up to 500 ml/min); in the latter site the hands show the most striking increase. As with cardiac output, most of the rise in extrauterine sites occurs during the first 10 weeks of pregnancy.

Endothelin

Endothelin is a 21-amino-acid peptide, secreted by endothelial cells, which has long-lasting vasoconstrictor activity. Maternal circulating levels increase during pregnancy. At delivery, fetal levels are higher than maternal and the highest levels are found in amniotic fluid.

Blood volume and composition

Plasma volume increases during pregnancy, reaching a plateau at 32–34 weeks. The increase is 1250 ml in a first pregnancy and 1500 ml in subsequent pregnancies (non-pregnant volume 2600 ml).

Red cell mass increases by 240 ml (400 ml for those given iron) (non-pregnant mass 1400 ml). Increased red cell production is probably stimulated by a three-fold rise in erythropoietin levels and is associated with an increase in the proportion of fetal haemoglobin (HbF). Blood loss at delivery averages 500 ml.

Changes in the cellular composition of the blood are shown in Table 3.1.

Haematinic factors in pregnancy

Iron

A normal diet contains 14 mg iron per day, of which 5%–10% (1–2 mg) is absorbed in the non-pregnant state and up to 40% during pregnancy. Iron must be converted to the ferrous form for absorption, a process which is enhanced by ascorbic acid and hydrochloric acid. Some foods (grains, eggs) contain iron complexed to phytates or phosphates, which decreases absorption. Iron requirements of pregnancy are shown in Table 3.2.

Table 3.1. Changes in cell composition of blood during pregnancy. Note that changes in cell factors are very dependent on iron supplementation

Component	Change
Total white cell count	Increase
Neutrophils	Increase[a]
Lymphocytes	No change
Eosinophils[c]	
Platelets	Decrease
Red cell count	Decrease
Haematocrit (packed cell volume)	Decrease
Haemoglobin concentration	Decrease[b]
Mean cell haemoglobin concentration	No change
Mean cell volume	Small increase
Red cell fragility	Increase
Erythrocyte sedimentation rate	Increase

[a] Metabolic activity and enzymes (e.g. alkaline phosphatase) also increase
[b] Acceptable minimum 11g/dl (WHO)
[c] Fall sharply during labour and delivery

Table 3.2. Iron requirements in pregnancy. Overall demand is 4 mg/day, being lower in early pregnancy and greater in late pregnancy. Normal women should receive a supplement of 30–60 mg/day.

	Iron (mg)
Increase in red cell mass	570
Normal loss (skin, urine, faeces)	270
Fetus	200-370
Placental/umbilical cord	35–50
Blood loss at delivery	100–250
Breast feeding	100–180
Total (approx.)	1200–1700
Less conservation due to amenorrhoea	240–480
Total (approx.)	700–1400

Serum iron (normal level 13–27 µmol/litre) decreases by 35% in pregnancy in the absence of full iron supplementation. Iron in plasma is bound to transferrin. Transferrin levels and hence iron-binding capacity are increased in pregnancy; this increase is not affected by iron supplements.

In tissues iron is stored with ferritin. Ferritin levels in blood, which reflect tissue iron stores, fall in early pregnancy but do not reach iron deficiency levels if iron supplements are given. Iron deficiency leads to a microcytic, hypochromic anaemia.

Folate

A normal Western diet contains 500–700 µg folic acid per day, of which 10%–100% may be lost in cooking. Requirements increase during pregnancy

(400–800 μg/day) and can be met by supplements of 200–300 μg/day. Folic acid absorbed from the diet is reduced in the tissues to the active form, tetrahydrofolic acid. Folate is actively transported by the placenta to the fetus, and the maternal plasma folate level falls by almost half during pregnancy (from 6 μg/litre to 3.5 μg/litre).

Folate deficiency may occur during pregnancy or the puerperium and leads to megaloblastic anaemia apparent in both blood films and bone marrow aspirates. Subclinical deficiency can be identified by measurement of folate in plasma or red cells, or by an increase in urinary excretion of formiminoglutamic acid after a loading dose of histidine. Folate supplementation reduces the frequency of neural tube defects.

Vitamin B_{12}

The requirement of 3 μg/day in pregnancy is met by any diet except strict vegetarian. Vitamin B_{12} is actively transported by the placenta to the fetus. Serum vitamin B_{12} levels fall during pregnancy, although the body stores are little affected and deficiency is rare.

Coagulation and fibrinolysis during pregnancy

Plasma levels of factors VII, VIII, IX, X and XII, together with fibrinogen and fibrin degradation products, increase during pregnancy (fibrinogen from 2.5–4 g/litre to 6 g/litre). Factor XI and antithrombin III levels decrease. These changes are consistent with a general increase in coagulability. Excessive intravascular coagulation and fibrinolysis are features of pathological conditions such as placental abruption and pre-eclampsia.

Fetal circulation

Cardiovascular system

The major variants in the fetal cardiovascular system are explained by the presence of the umbilical–placental circulation and the absence of a significant pulmonary circulation. The pathway of fetal blood is summarised in Fig. 3.1. High venous return from the placenta maintains the right–left shunt through the foramen ovale and delivers the most oxygenated blood to the brain and heart. Oxygen saturation is 70%–80% in the umbilical vein and ductus venosus and 60% in the left atrium. Blood entering the right atrium from the inferior vena cava tends to be directed through the foramen ovale into the left atrium, while deoxygenated blood entering from the superior vena cava is directed towards the right ventricle. Most of the latter stream will enter the systemic circulation via the ductus arteriosus and is thereby diverted to the descending aorta, while the brain receives a greater proportion of the oxygenated blood from the left side of the heart. High pulmonary vascular resistance maintains the right–left shunt through the ductus arteriosus. The right ventricle has slightly higher cardiac output than the left ventricle, and over three-quarters of this is shunted into the systemic circulation.

Fetal cardiac output is relatively greater than adult cardiac output (100 $ml \cdot kg^{-1} \cdot min^{-1}$ per ventricle vs 80 $ml \cdot kg^{-1} \cdot min^{-1}$ per ventricle) and is mainly determined by heart rate under the control of the autonomic nervous system. Nevertheless, the fetal heart obeys Starling's Law and an increased end-diastolic volume (e.g. after an extrasystole) results in a larger stroke volume. The proportion of the cardiac output directed to the placenta decreases from 50% at mid-pregnancy to 40% by term. This does not change during hypoxia, but blood-flow to the adrenals, brain and heart is increased while that to the kidney is decreased. The umbilical arterial blood-flow (100–120 $ml \cdot kg^{-1} \cdot min^{-1}$) is relatively high

Umbilical vein
↓
Ductus venosus
↓
Inferior vena cava
↓
Right atrium
↓
Foramen ovale
↓
Left atrium
↓
Left ventricle
↓
Ascending aorta
↓
Coronary/cerebral arteries
↓
Superior vena cava
↓
Right atrium
↓
Right ventricle
↓
Pulmonary artery   (10% lung)
↓
Ductus arteriosus
↓
Descending aorta
↓
Umbilical artery

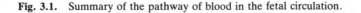

Fig. 3.1. Summary of the pathway of blood in the fetal circulation.

during diastole, indicating a low-resistance circulation, as demonstrated by Doppler bloodflow studies. Fetal blood pressure is 40–60 mmHg.

At birth the cessation of umbilical blood-flow causes a fall in pressure in the right atrium and closure of the foramen ovale. Ventilation of the lungs opens the pulmonary circulation and the ductus arteriosus closes as a direct effect of increasing Po_2. Prior to birth the ductus remains patent due to production of prostaglandin E_2 and prostacyclin, which act as local vasodilators.

Factors affecting fetal heart rate

Fetal heart rate (FHR) falls progressively after 9 weeks. Before 32 weeks the range is 160–180 beats/min. By term it is in the range 120–160 beats/min. Beat-to-beat variation (5 beats/min) and sensitivity to ganglion-stimulating drugs develop after the 20th week. Compression of the head or neck produces a transient bradycardia; compression of the thorax or abdomen results in a transient tachycardia. Bradycardia may occur when the mother defecates, urinates or vomits during labour. Increases in fetal heart rate may accompany fetal movements, sound and vibration, and maternal anxiety.

Fetal blood

The first blood cells are formed in 'blood islands' on the surface of the yolk sac. During the 6th week of embryonic life, extramedullary haemopoiesis begins in the liver and to a lesser extent in the spleen. These sites are maximally developed at 16 weeks, when the bone marrow starts to produce red cells.

Most haemoglobin in the fetus is HbF, which has two γ-chains (α-2, γ-2), in place of the adult haemoglobins HbA (α-2, β-2) and HbA2 (α-2, δ-2). γ-Chains are made by two genes which make two slightly different forms of γ-chain, while β-chains are identical and come from a single gene. β, γ and δ genes are on chromosome 11. HbF is resistant to denaturation by acid and alkali and has a higher affinity for oxygen than adult haemoglobin in vivo. Ninety per cent of fetal haemoglobin is HbF between 10 and 28 weeks of gestation. From 28 to 34 weeks a switch from (α-2, γ-2) to (α-2, β-2) begins. By term the ratio of HbF to HbA is 80 : 20, and by 6 months only 1% of haemoglobin is HbF. In the normal adult less than 1% of haemoglobin is HbF. Between 4 and 8 weeks the embryo manufactures some additional haemoglobins: Hb Gower 1 (ϵ- and ζ-chains), Hb Gower 2 (α- and ζ-chains) and Hb Portland (ϵ- and γ-chains).

Fetal red cells are larger than maternal cells and possess the i antigen, which is replaced by the I antigen after birth. They are more resistant than adult cells to osmotic alkali and acid lysis, have a shorter life span, and have lower levels of 2,3-diphosphoglyceric acid and carbonic anhydrase. Fetal cells have no surface ABO antigen until after birth.

At birth the mean capillary haemoglobin level is 18 g%. The capillary venous difference is larger than in older children and averages 3.5 g%; the difference is further enhanced in anaemia and prematurity.

Lung

Measurement of lung function

The meaning of terms commonly used to describe lung function are summarised in Table 3.3 and standard tests of ventilation in Table 3.4.

Changes in lung function during pregnancy

During pregnancy the diaphragm rises 4 cm, the transverse diameter of the chest increases by 2 cm and the subcostal angle increases from 68° to 103°. The

Table 3.3. Terms commonly used to describe the function of the lung (approximate non-pregnant value in parentheses)

Term	Meaning
Tidal volume	Volume of air inspired or expired in each respiration (500 ml)
Inspiratory reserve volume	Maximum amount of air which can be inspired beyond normal tidal volume (3000 ml)
Expiratory reserve volume	Maximum amount of air which can be expired from the resting end-expiratory position (1100 ml)
Residual volume	Volume of air in lungs after maximal expiration (excluding bronchi and trachea) (1200 ml)
Alveolar ventilation	Tidal volume minus dead space (bronchi/trachea/non-functioning alveoli)
Total lung capacity	Amount of air in lung after maximal inspiration
Vital capacity	Inspiratory reserve volume + tidal volume + expiratory reserve volume (4600 ml)
Functional residual capacity	Amount of air remaining in the resting end-expiratory position (2300 ml)
Minute volume	Amount of air inspired in a minute (7.5 litres/min)

Table 3.4. Standard tests of lung function

Test	Description
Maximum breathing capacity	Maximum amount of air which can be inspired or expired by forced voluntary breathing over 15 s
Forced expiratory volume in one second	Amount of air which can be forcibly expired from maximal inspiration in 1 s
Peak expiratory flow rate	Maximum rate of air-flow during forced expiration (measured with Wright peak flow meter)

Table 3.5. Changes in lung function during pregnancy (extent of change is shown in parentheses)

Test	Change
Respiratory rate	No change
Vital capacity	Increase in some but not all subjects
Inspiratory capacity	Increase (300 ml)
Expiratory reserve volume	Decrease (200 ml)
Residual volume	Decrease (300 ml)
Functional residual capacity	Decrease (500 ml)
Tidal volume	Increase (200 ml)
Minute ventilation	Increase (3 litres/min)
Maximum breathing capacity	No change
Forced expiratory volume	No change

increase in overall breathing (see below) is primarily the result of increased diaphragmatic excursion.

The changes in lung function during pregnancy are summarised in Table 3.5 and Fig. 3.2. Overall, there is an increase in ventilation attributed to a greater depth of breathing but not to an increase in rate. The prime stimulus to this is the increase in circulating progesterone levels.

Oxygen consumption increases during pregnancy from 250 ml/min to 300 ml/min. Because this 20% increase is less than the 50% for alveolar ventilation, there is an effective 'hyperventilation', and both alveolar and arterial P_{CO_2} are reduced (35–40 mmHg in non-pregnant; 30 mmHg in

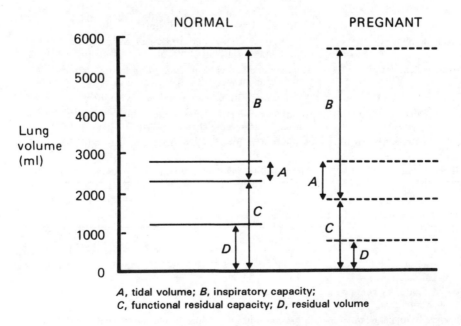

A, tidal volume; B, inspiratory capacity;
C, functional residual capacity; D, residual volume

Fig. 3.2. Changes in lung function during pregnancy.

pregnancy). This, in turn, leads to a reduction in plasma bicarbonate and sodium, and hence in osmolality. Arterial pH is unchanged. Arterial P_{CO_2} shows a small increase.

Fetal lung

The lung forms as an outgrowth of the primitive foregut, and full differentiation of capillary and canalicular elements is apparent by the 20th week. Alveoli develop after 24 weeks. Numerous but intermittent fetal breathing movements occur in utero, especially during REM sleep or periods of hypoxia. Fetal breathing occurs for 15% of the observation time in the second trimester rising to 30% in the third trimester. Time spent breathing increases after meals and decreases after alcohol ingestion and during labour.

Lung alveoli are lined by a group of phospholipids known collectively as surfactant. Surfactant prevents collapse of small alveoli during expiration by lowering surface tension[1] or by acting as an internal molecular 'splint'. The surfactant is continually replaced by synthesis from type II alveolar cells. These cells make up 10% of the lung parenchyma. Surfactant is produced on microsomes and stored in 1.5 μm osmiophilic lamellar bodies.

The predominant phospholipid (80% of total) is dipalmitoylphosphatidylcholine (DPPC; lecithin). There is a surge of lecithin production at 35–36 weeks of fetal life. The surge can be promoted by cortisol, growth retardation and prolonged rupture of the membranes, and is delayed in diabetes. Before this pathway is activated, the lung is functionally immature, and premature delivery is often associated with respiratory distress syndrome (RDS). Surfactant is associated with a group of proteins which enhances activity.

Other phospholipids included in surfactant are sphingomyelin, phosphatidyl glycerol and phosphatidyl inositol. Sphingomyelin production reaches a peak at about 32 weeks and diminishes after 35 weeks. Some lung liquid is excreted into amniotic fluid and the lecithin:sphingomyelin ratio in this site therefore provides a measure of lung maturity. The action of lecithin is dependent on phosphatidyl inositol (secreted early in the second trimester) and phosphatidyl glycerol (secreted mainly in the last 5 weeks of pregnancy). The relative deficiency of phosphatidyl glycerol in diabetic pregnancies may lead to the development of RDS despite a 'mature' lecithin:sphingomyelin ratio (more than 2).

Fetal asphyxia during labour is associated with variation in fetal heart rate (normal 120–160/min), including: (a) variable or late decelerations, (b) baseline tachycardia, and (c) loss of beat-to-beat variability (normal ±5 beats/min). Scalp blood pH falls because of lactic acid accumulation (normal >7.25; borderline asphyxia 7.2–7.25; definitive asphyxia <7.2). The pH of fetal blood also falls in the presence of respiratory acidosis.

---

[1] This effect is described by Laplace's law:
$$p = 2T/r$$
where p = pressure, T = surface tension and r = radius. Thus small alveoli would generate high pressure and empty into the larger alveoli if their surface tension was not reduced.

The fetus has a large capacity for anaerobic metabolism and can withstand asphyxia better than the adult in the presence of adequate glycogen reserves.

Fetal blood-gas status during pregnancy

In umbilical blood there is a progressive decrease in Po_2 from 16 to 40 weeks and an increase in Pco_2, bicarbonate, base excess and lactate.

The first breath – commencement of breathing at birth

At delivery, commencement of breathing is stimulated by: (a) rising carbon dioxide levels and acidosis, (b) change in thermal and tactile stimuli, (c) thoracic compression in the vagina, and (d) general changes in level of arousal. Breathing should commence within 20–30 s; a delay of more than 1 min is an indication for assistance.

Aeration is accomplished by inspiration and clearance of lung fluid. A negative intrathoracic pressure of −20 to −70 cmH$_2$O is required to achieve this, together with a positive expiratory pressure of 20–30 cmH$_2$O associated with expiration against a closed glottis.

Acid–base balance

The pH is the reciprocal of the logarithm of the hydrogen ion (H$^+$) concentration. A pH of 7 represents neutrality and at this point both the H$^+$ and OH$^-$ concentrations are 100 nEq/litre.

The normal pH of arterial blood is 7.4 (H$^+$ 40 nEq/litre) and that of venous blood and interstitial fluid is 7.35; intracellular pH averages 7.0. All body fluids contain buffer systems, which respond to and correct small pH changes in fractions of a second. Blood pH is controlled by the lungs and kidneys.

The main buffer system controlling blood pH is carbonic acid/sodium bicarbonate (in cells, potassium and magnesium bicarbonate). The usual ratio of bicarbonate to carbonic acid is 20:1. The pH can be described by the Henderson–Hasselbalch equation:

$$pH = pK + \log \frac{HCO_3^-}{H_2CO_3}$$

The pK is a constant (6.1), defining the H$_2$CO$_3$/HCO$_3^-$ buffer system. The body normally deals with an acid load more efficiently than an alkaline load. The excess H$^+$ ions bind to HCO$_3^-$ to form H$_2$CO$_3$ and this in turn

Table 3.6. Clinical abnormalities of acid–base balance. The main effect of acidosis is depression of the central nervous system (disorientation, coma). The main effect of alkalosis is over-excitability of the central nervous system (tetany). Note that a respiratory abnormality will stimulate a compensatory metabolic response, and vice versa.

Type of disturbance	Mechanism	Causes
Respiratory acidosis	Increase of blood CO_2 owing to inadequate lung ventilation	Breath holding, brain damage and any disease which reduces ventilation or gas exchange in the lungs
Respiratory alkalosis	Decrease of blood CO_2 owing to excessive lung ventilation	Overbreathing (psychiatric disorders, pregnancy, high altitudes)
Metabolic acidosis	Excess of fixed acids (i.e. everything except CO_2)	Renal failure, loss of alkali (diarrhoea and vomiting, diabetes mellitus, carbonic anhydrase inhibitors, elevated extracellular potassium, the fetus in fetal distress)
Metabolic alkalosis	Deficiency of fixed acids	Diuretic therapy, excess bicarbonate ingestion (ulcers), gastric vomiting, excess aldosterone

dissociates to water and carbon dioxide (99.9% is in the form of dissolved CO_2 and only 0.1% as H_2CO_3). The concentration of carbon dioxide in blood (normal 1.2 mmol/litre) controls the respiratory centre in the medulla oblongata and hence the rate of breathing and the elimination of carbon dioxide (a response which takes 1–15 min). Neutralisation of hydrogen ions and elimination of carbon dioxide will also reduce the amount of bicarbonate. This is replenished by the proximal convoluted tubule, in which carbonic anhydrase catalyses the reaction

$$CO_2 + H_2O \rightarrow H_2CO_3 \rightarrow HCO_3^- + H^+$$

The bicarbonate is secreted into the blood and hydrogen ions into the urine. The renal response to acid–base changes is relatively slow (hours or days).

Other buffer systems in the body include (a) the phosphate buffer system ($H_2PO_4^-/HPO_4^{2-}$), which is important inside cells and in the kidney tubules, and (b) the protein buffer system, which is also a key intracellular factor.

Clinical abnormalities of acid–base balance

Clinical abnormalities of acid–base balance are summarised in Table 3.6. Maternal respiratory acidosis is transmitted to the fetus, as the excess carbon dioxide can cross the placenta. Metabolic acidosis has less effect as the placenta is not permeable to hydrogen ions. The concentration and buffering action of bicarbonate in the fetus is relatively lower than that in the adult.

Kidney

The kidneys enlarge during pregnancy (1 cm in length) and there is dilatation of the collecting system, including the calyces, renal pelvis and ureters in 90% of women. These changes occur from the first trimester and are more prominent on the right side (compression by dilated left ovarian vein). Causes may include ureteric obstruction at the pelvic brim.

Renal blood-flow (effective renal plasma-flow) increases 70%–80% by mid-pregnancy; during the third trimester it decreases but is still 50%–60% above non-pregnancy levels. Glomerular filtration (as measured by clearance of creatinine, inulin, p-aminohippurate or iohexol) increases by 30%–50% during pregnancy, beginning in the first 2 weeks of pregnancy. As a result plasma levels of creatinine and urea fall: the upper limits of normal in late pregnancy are 75 μmol/litre and 4.5 mmol/litre respectively. Clearance of uric acid is also increased, but this is balanced by increased tubular reabsorption, and in late pregnancy the plasma levels are similar to those in the non-pregnant state.

Renal excretion of a variety of materials during pregnancy is increased owing to an increase in filtered load which is greater than tubular reabsorptive capacity. Such materials include glucose and other sugars, water-soluble vitamins, serum proteins (including albumin and transferrin) and amino acids.

Renal acid–base regulation (bicarbonate absorption and acid (H^+) excretion) is unchanged during pregnancy. There is a slight retention of potassium (total 350 mEq). Although plasma osmolality is reduced (by 10 mosmol/kg), vasopressin (AVP, antidiuretic hormone) levels are normal, presumably owing to resetting of osmoreceptors. The ability to excrete a water load is subject to marked postural effects, being greater in the lateral recumbent than in either the supine or the upright position. This may be the result of compression of the renal veins by the gravid uterus. Similarly, the creatinine clearance is higher at night, in contrast to the non-pregnant state.

Cumulative water retention in pregnancy is 7.5 litres and this is accompanied by 900 mmol sodium. The increase in filtered load of sodium (from 20 000 mmol/day to 30 000 mmol/day) is balanced by greater tubular reabsorption. This pattern is influenced by a variety of hormones, most notably the sodium-retaining steroids aldosterone and deoxycorticosterone (DOC), both of which increase during pregnancy. The increased aldosterone results, at least in part, from the elevated plasma concentrations of renin. Angiotensin I and II are also substantially increased and pregnant women are highly resistant to the pressor effects of infused angiotensin II. The uterus and amniotic fluid contain high levels of renin-like material.

Fetal urine flow is greater during active (REM) sleep than in quiet (non-REM) sleep.

Nervous system

Fetal hearing commences at 26–28 weeks gestation. High-frequency sounds (above 250 Hz) are attenuated by maternal tissues.

Gut and nutrition

Appetite

Appetite and thirst increase during pregnancy. Inability to take large meals
in late pregnancy leads to more frequent eating of snacks. Food aversions
or preferences may develop associated with a reduction in the sense of taste.
There is an increase in the levels of both motilin and somatostatin throughout
pregnancy.

Changes in the maternal gastrointestinal system during pregnancy

Many of these changes can be ascribed to the relaxation of smooth muscle
under the influence of progesterone.

Gums, teeth and saliva.   The gums may swell due to oedema and bleed easily.
The incidence of caries is increased. Secretion of saliva (1–2 litres/day) is
usually unchanged.

Oesophagus and stomach.   Reduced competence of the lower oesophageal
sphincter may lead to reflux oesophagitis.
    Gastric secretion of both acid and peptide enzymes is reduced in mid-
pregnancy. Gastric tone and motility are also reduced, especially during
labour, and the emptying time is increased from 50 min to 100 min.

The intestines.   Both the small and the large intestine have reduced motility
during pregnancy.

The liver and gall bladder.   Most standard liver function tests are normal
in pregnancy; the fall in plasma albumin (a dilutional effect) and rise in
heat-labile serum alkaline phosphatase (increased osteoclastic activity) do
not reflect disordered liver function.
    Dye clearance (e.g. bromsulphthalein) is less rapid than usual in pregnancy,
probably because of increased levels of binding proteins in blood. Serum bile
acids (cholylglycine) rise during pregnancy.
    Gall bladder motility and emptying rate are reduced in pregnancy.

Fetal gut

The fetal gut differentiates from endoderm by 6 weeks after conception.
Swallowing movements are present by 14 weeks and a full sucking reflex

Table 3.7. Average weight gain attributable to various sources at 40 weeks gestation

Tissue/fluid	Gain (kg)
Fetus	3400
Placenta	650
Amniotic fluid	800
Uterus	970
Mammary gland	400
Blood	1250
Extracellular extravascular fluid	1700
Fat	3500

by 28 weeks. Secretion of bile and digestive enzymes begins at 12 weeks. Meconium is present by 16 weeks and consists of desquamated intestinal cells, intestinal juices and squamous cells.

Maternal nutrition during pregnancy

The total extra requirement (mother and fetus) for protein during pregnancy is about 900 g. Only 70% of high-grade dietary protein is usable for protein stores, this figure being lower with certain diets such as those based on cassava. Much of the excess protein requirement occurs in late pregnancy and at this time the mother needs an extra 8.5 g/day of dietary protein to remain in balance.

The total requirement for fat during pregnancy is 3.5 kg, most of which occurs during the second and early third trimester. The cumulative net energy cost of maintaining the fetus and added maternal tissues is 80 000 kcal. The extra energy required in the last weeks of pregnancy is 250 kcal/day (about one-quarter of non-pregnant expenditure). In normal women this is provided by dietary increase (200 kcal/day) and reduced activity.

The extra requirement for calcium is 30 mg, for sodium 950 mEq (approx. 40 mg) and for potassium 320 mEq (8 mg).

Maternal weight gain during pregnancy

Maternal weight gain averages 0.35 kg/week in early pregnancy, 0.45 kg/week in mid-pregnancy and 0.35 kg/week in late pregnancy. The average total weight gain is 12.5 kg. The contributions to this gain from identified sources are shown in Table 3.7.

Fetal weight gain during pregnancy

The weight of the fetus at delivery is related to the height and weight of the mother but not the father. Women of Indian, African and Chinese origin have smaller babies than European women. First babies are smaller (by 100 g) than subsequent babies. Fetal genotype determines fetal size in early pregnancy; maternal factors are apparent only towards the end of pregnancy. Fetal weight at term is related to maternal weight gain during pregnancy. It is lower in smokers than in non-smokers, in pregnancies at high altitude, in mothers with chronic anaemia and in drug addicts. Growth of the fetus is not affected by maternal diet unless there is extreme deprivation. Most of the variation in fetal weight at term is accounted for by body fat.

Metabolism

Energy comes from carbohydrate (4.4 kcal/g), protein (4.2 kcal/g) and fat (7 kcal/g). The body stores these after a meal and mobilises them for metabolism on demand. Glycogen is the first resource, followed by fat. Protein is used only in extreme starvation or in shock states.

Carbohydrate metabolism

Glucose is immediately phosphorylated in cells by hexokinase to glucose 6-phosphate. It is then converted to glycogen, metabolised by anaerobic glycolysis or metabolised by the pentose shunt.

Anaerobic glycolysis is a means by which glucose provides:

1. Energy (in the form of ATP) – this is the sole source of energy under anaerobic conditions, e.g. in muscles during strenuous exercise

2. Pyruvate for aerobic glycolysis (Fig. 3.3)

3. Acetyl coenzyme A (acetyl CoA) for production of fat when energy intake exceeds energy expenditure

Glycolysis of one molecule of glucose yields two molecules of ATP, and two molecules of nicotinamide adenine dinucleotide (NAD) are reduced to NADH.

The pentose shunt is aerobic (oxygen is consumed and carbon dioxide produced). It is active in many tissues (e.g. fat and red blood cells) and leads to reduction of nicotinamide adenine nucleotide phosphate (NADP) to NADPH. This pathway provides the pentose (five carbon) sugars essential for nucleic acid synthesis.

The tricarboxylic acid (Krebs or citric acid) cycle involves oxidation of several substrates and is a major source of ATP and carbon dioxide. Four molecules of NAD are reduced during each cycle to produce NADH and $FADH_2$ (from flavin adenine dinucleotide, FAD). One molecule of NADH is also produced from the conversion of pyruvate to acetyl CoA. Each of the reduced nucleotides may be oxidised in mitochondria to produce two to three molecules of ATP. Because two pyruvate molecules are produced from each glucose molecule and the glycolytic pathway yields a net of two molecules of ATP per molecule of glucose, the complete oxidation of a glucose molecule yields 32 molecules of ATP.

Lipid metabolism

Ninety per cent of glucose is converted and stored as fat. Fatty acid synthesis takes place in adipose tissue and to a lesser extent in the liver. Fatty acids are derived from acetyl CoA (Fig. 3.3). Several reductions of NADH, NADPH and FADH are required. This pathway is reversible so that fat may be metabolised in times of need.

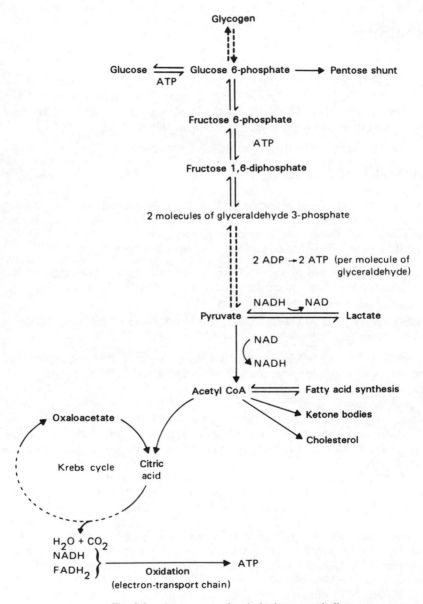

Fig. 3.3. A summary of carbohydrate metabolism.

Endocrine control of energy metabolism

Energy metabolism is controlled by insulin, glucagon, adrenaline, cortisol, thyroxine, growth hormone and placental lactogen.

Pancreatic islets

The β cells of the pancreas secrete insulin; α cells make glucagon and the δ cells somatostatin. Of islet cells, 60%–80% are β cells and 20%–30% are α cells.

Insulin

Insulin (mol. wt. 4500) consists of two chains of amino acids joined by three disulphide bonds. The molecule is derived from a larger precursor, pro-insulin; cleavage prior to release yields insulin and the C-peptide, which are secreted in equimolar amounts. Insulin has a half-life of about 10 min. In the liver and placenta the disulphide bonds are reduced by glutathione insulin transhydrogenase to yield A and B fragments.

Insulin has the following effects:

1. Hypoglycaemia due to (a) decreased glucose production by the liver and (b) increased peripheral uptake by some tissues, particularly fat and muscle. The CNS (except the ventromedial satiety centre in the hypothalamus), liver, intestine, kidney, islets of Langerhans and placenta do not require insulin for glucose entry.

2. Promotion of glycogen synthesis.

3. Depression of gluconeogenesis from alanine and other glucogenic amino acids.

4. Promotion of amino acid transport into liver and muscle.

5. Promotion of free fatty acid synthesis from acetyl CoA.

6. Inhibition of glucagon secretion.

7. Enhancement of fetal growth. This is the mechanism of macrosomia in diabetic mothers; maternal hyperglycaemia leads to fetal hyperinsulinaemia. Insulin does not cross the placenta. However, if the mother has antibodies to insulin, the insulin–antibody complex can cross the placenta and cause macrosomia even when the maternal blood sugar level is normal.

Glucagon

Glucagon is a single-chain polypeptide (mol. wt. 3500) with a similar half-life to that of insulin. It is a powerful hyperglycaemic agent, acting rapidly by mobilising liver glycogen and more slowly by stimulating gluconeogenesis. In addition it increases lipolysis, stimulates insulin and catecholamine release, and has bronchodilator and positive inotropic effects.

Control of insulin and glucagon

The following factors are involved:

1. Glucose stimulates release of insulin and inhibits glucagon secretion by a direct action on islets.

2. Amino acids, especially leucine, stimulate release of both insulin and glucagon.

3. Insulin inhibits glucagon release and glucagon stimulates insulin release.

4. Various gastrointestinal hormones stimulate insulin secretion (thus glucose levels are higher after intravenous infusion than after oral administration of glucose).

5. β-Adrenergic stimulation increases insulin output (e.g. exercise).

Hormones and metabolism

Insulin is the only hypoglycaemic hormone, whereas glucagon, adrenaline, growth hormone, cortisol, thyroxine and placental lactogen all increase blood sugar levels and are stimulated by hypoglycaemia. If the blood glucose concentration falls below 3.3 mmol/litre (60 mg/100 ml), insulin secretion ceases altogether: no glucose can enter muscle and fat cells, which then depend on fat for energy. Thus glucose is spared for the nervous system, which depends exclusively on glucose as an energy source.

Maternal and fetal metabolism during pregnancy

Carbohydrates

In pregnancy the action of insulin is blunted; this unmasks latent diabetes and aggravates existing diabetes. The non-diabetic mother has slightly lower than normal blood glucose levels and higher than normal insulin levels. However, the 2 h plasma glucose level after an oral glucose load increases during pregnancy. This is associated with an enhanced insulin response to glucose, which is apparent early in the second trimester, increases throughout pregnancy and disappears within 1 or 2 days of delivery. During fasting, insulin levels fall to those in the non-pregnant state, but all the normal adaptations to starvation are triggered more rapidly and more severely. Maternal fatty acid levels are higher during pregnancy.

The factors that promote glucose production during pregnancy include:

1. Human placental lactogen (hPL), which has a growth-hormone-like effect.

2. Oestrogens, which antagonise the peripheral actions of insulin.

3. Increased body mass, which increases the requirement for insulin.

4. A small increase in free cortisol.

Prior to the establishment of the circulation, the fetus derives energy by glycolysis alone. The Krebs cycle becomes important after the establishment of the circulation (day 21 of embryonic life).

Protein

The total protein, albumin and colloid osmotic pressure of serum fall abruptly in the first trimester and more slowly thereafter. Total globulin concentration rises, including specific increases in binding proteins, transferrin, specific pregnancy proteins and IgM; IgG levels decrease.

The fetus synthesises protein from amino acids derived by placental transfer.

Lipids

There is a general increase in plasma lipid levels during pregnancy, including triglycerides, cholesterol, phospholipids, non-esterified (i.e. free) fatty acids and lipoproteins (all classes). There is some evidence that the rise may be preceded by a fall in the first trimester.

Unlike the situation in the adult, fatty acids are not a significant energy source for the fetus. Fetal tissues can synthesise fatty acids, triglycerides, phospholipids and cholesterol. This, together with maternal sources, provides for the deposition of adipose tissue, which takes place during the last 6–10 weeks of pregnancy.

Amino acids

Maternal plasma concentrations of most amino acids fall during pregnancy. Fetal blood levels of amino acids are generally higher than maternal blood levels.

Vitamins

There are rises in plasma concentrations of carotenoids (provitamin A) and tocopherol (vitamin E), and reductions in retinol (vitamin A), ascorbic acid (vitamin C), folate, vitamin B_{12}, vitamin B_6, biotin, thiamine (vitamin B_1), riboflavine and nicotinic acid. Those showing a rise are in the fat-soluble group; the increased renal excretion causes a fall in levels of water-soluble vitamins. Fetal levels of water-soluble vitamins are generally higher than maternal levels.

Calcium

Some 30 g of calcium are incorporated into the fetus by term, mostly in the second half of pregnancy. This is associated with reductions in maternal plasma total calcium and magnesium (ionised calcium and phosphate are unchanged), and increased absorption of dietary calcium associated with an increase in 1,25-dihydroxycholecalciferol (calcitriol) and parathormone. Extra requirements of calcium and vitamin D can be met by a normal diet, although some women of Asian origin may require vitamin D supplements.

Fetal plasma concentrations of calcium and phosphate are greater than maternal plasma concentrations because of active placental transport.

Trace metals

1. *Zinc*: Maternal blood levels of zinc decrease during pregnancy. Zinc concentrations in umbilical blood are higher than maternal levels.

2. *Copper*: Maternal serum copper concentrations increase 2–3 times above that in the non-pregnant state, associated with an increase in caeruloplasmin levels. Umbilical blood copper concentration is one-eighth that of maternal blood.

Immunology

General immunology

Non-specific factors

Non-specific defences include phagocytosis, lysozyme, several of the mediators of the inflammatory response (e.g. kinins) and lymphokines. Lymphokines are responsible for molecular signalling between cells of the immune system. Because they can be produced to some extent by all cells, they are also known as 'cytokines'. Lymphokines include the interleukins, tumour necrosis factor, colony stimulating factors and the interferons. An interferon is a naturally occurring glycoprotein which protects against viral infection. Its action is dependent on combination with a cell surface receptor, which leads to intracellular inhibition of the nucleic acid production on which viral replication depends. It also affects host cell DNA replication, and human interferon has some anti-tumour activity. It is produced by leucocytes (α-interferon) of which there are 12 subtypes, fibroblasts (β-interferon) and lymphocytes (γ-interferon). Relatively high levels of α-interferon are found in amniotic fluid, the placenta and other fetal tissues.

Cellular immunity

Specific immunity depends on lymphocytes, which arise from stem cells in bone marrow and are of two major groups: B cells, which are precursors of plasma cells and secrete specific antibody; and T cells, which mature in the thymus and are involved with cell-mediated immunity. T cells are of three main types: (a) cytotoxic T cells (natural killer (NK) cells), which directly kill foreign or virus-infected cells; (b) T-helper cells, which assist B cells in the antibody response, and other T cells in cell-mediated responses; (c) T-suppressor cells, which inhibit the responses of B cells and other T cells. T-helper and T-suppressor cells act chiefly by secretion of lymphokines.

T cells recognise foreign antigens via a surface receptor. This is activated only when the antigen is associated with cell-membrane glycoprotein of the major histocompatibility complex (MHC), a group of proteins coded by 40–50 genes on chromosome 6. There are two classes of MHC proteins: (a) class I, expressed on most cells and which in humans include the HLA (human leucocyte antigen) system (HLA-A, B, C, E, F and G); (b) class II, (DP, DQ and DR antigens) expressed on B cells, some T cells and macrophages.

Antigen processing cells (APCs; monocytes, macrophages, histiocytes, dendritic cells) play a key role in the immune response. Antigen–antibody complexes adhere to the APC surface and stimulate all types of T cell.

The B cell responses are initiated by reaction between antigen and an immunoglobulin receptor on the cell surface. B cells proliferate and mature into plasma cells. Individual clones of B cells secrete antibodies of unique specificity. Many clones are involved in an immune response and the serum therefore contains antibodies of multiple specificities.

Antibodies

The general structure of the antibody (immunoglobulin) molecule is shown in Fig. 3.4. There are four main classes of immunoglobulin (Table 3.8), each with a distinctive heavy (H) chain.

The primary response follows initial exposure to an antigen and results in antibody production after about 10 days. Thereafter the stimulated clones of lymphocytes persist at a lower level of activity, providing the 'memory' which will enable a much more rapid response to re-exposure.

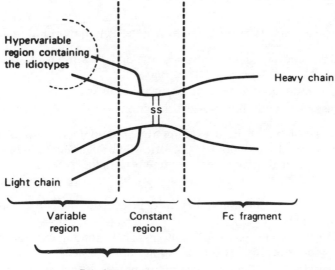

Fig. 3.4. The IgG molecule. The N-terminal 110 amino acids of the heavy (H) and light (L) chains are variable regions, which in turn contain three hypervariable regions that form the antigen-binding site. Each site is itself an antigen or 'idiotype' and there are as many idiotypes as antibody specificities. An immune response can thus lead to further anti-idiotype response, a process thought to play an important role in the control of immune reactions.

Table 3.8. Immunoglobulin classes. All B cells initially make IgM but can subsequently switch to other classes.

Class	Features
IgG (four subclasses, 1–4)	Molecular weight 160 000. Main immunoglobulin in plasma. Placenta has receptors; crosses to the fetus.
IgM	Molecular weight 900 000. Produced before IgG in the primary immune response but does not persist.
IgE	Binds to mast cells and basophils. Subsequent exposure to specific antigen causes type I allergic reactions such as anaphylaxis and urticaria. Involved in protection against helminthic infection.
IgA	Provides surface protection on mucous membranes. Secreted by local lymphoid tissue. Paired molecules acquire a glycoprotein 'secretory piece' which protects the secretory IgA from breakdown on epithelial surfaces.

Combination of antibody with antigen is seldom adequate as a defence mechanism on its own. However, the 'immune complex' so formed activates the complement system, which provides effective mechanisms. The complement system involves a 'cascade' of activating factors (Fig. 3.5). It may be initiated by antigen–antibody complexes (the classical pathway) or directly by endotoxin (the alternative pathway).

Changes in the immune system in pregnancy

Immunological changes in pregnancy are relatively minor and include:

1. Total leucocyte count increased by 30% owing to an increase in neutrophils. The lymphocyte count is unchanged.

2. A slight reduction in IgG and an increase in IgD.

3. Increased susceptibility to some infections (polio, influenza, malaria).

None of the above changes explains the immunological tolerance of the fetus and placenta by the mother. Theories that might explain why the fetus and placenta, which display paternal antigens from the 6–8 cell stage onwards, are not rejected in the same manner as any foreign organ graft are:

1. The uterus is an immunologically privileged site, like the anterior chamber of the eye.

2. Fetal antigens are 'blocked' by non-specific coating substances such as fibrinogen and mucoproteins on the trophoblast surface.

3. Immunoglobulins protect antigenic sites from attack by cytotoxic cells.

4. Blood group antigens and class I and II MHC are absent on the syncytiotrophoblast although class I HLA-G may be found on the extravillous trophoblast. Maternal antibodies to fetal HLA components are the result of transplacental passage of sensitising cells.

5. Local immunosuppression by placental proteins such as SP1 or PP14.

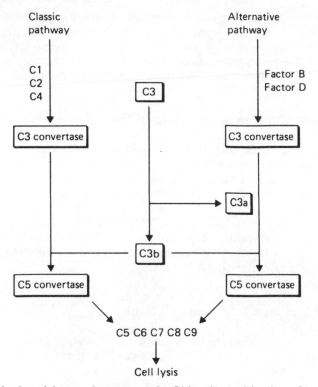

Fig. 3.5. Activation of the complement cascade. C1 has three subfractions, C1q, C1r and C1s; C1q binds the Fc of IgG or IgM. The central component is C3. The activated form C3b can bind to organisms and render them susceptible to phagocytosis; C3b also initiates the formation of a large lytic complex (the 'attack complex', C5b-9) in membranes, which can kill cells. In addition, a variety of small peptides are produced that attract leucocytes (C5a) and stimulate release of histamine from mast cells (C3a).

6. The stroma of the decidua contains large numbers of a unique type of large granular leucocyte, which are thought to be immunosuppressive.

A degree of maternal–paternal incompatibility may be important for a satisfactory pregnancy. Compatibility for HLA-DR antigens between husband and wife is associated with an increased incidence of abortion, growth retardation and major congenital anomalies.

Transfer of antibodies to the fetus

IgG (especially subclasses 1, 2 and 3) is transferred to the fetus during pregnancy by an active process, which is dependent on binding of the Fc part of the molecule to a specific placental receptor prior to endocytosis. This applies equally to endogenous and exogenous IgG. Maternal IgG can be transferred across the placenta from 6 weeks onwards. At term, fetal IgG level is 5%–10% greater than maternal. Other classes of immunoglobulins are not transferred. Neonatal thyrotoxicosis, myasthenia gravis and autoimmune thrombocytopenia may result from transfer of IgG, even after clinical remission in the mother. The antibodies of lupus erythematosus do little harm to the fetus, although occasionally they may cause temporary congenital heart block. Patients with the rare lupus anticoagulant in their serum may suffer abortion or intrauterine death due to obstruction of the placental circulation.

Development of the immune system in the fetus

The first haemopoietic centres develop in the yolk sac after 4 weeks of embryonic life and lymphocytes (T cells) develop in the thymus at about 8 weeks. At 12 weeks the liver and spleen produce B lymphocytes, and from this time onwards the fetus can recognise foreign antigens and reject allografts. However, most antibody is derived by active transfer from the mother.

At birth the lymphocyte count is 3000–5000/ml, increasing still further during the first week of life. The ratio of T to B cells is the same as in the adult (3:1). The neutrophil count increases to about 20 000 during the first day of life but thereafter slowly decreases.

Immunological aspects of amniotic fluid

Immunoglobulins are present from about 12 weeks and these, together with other specific antibacterial proteins (some containing zinc), have considerable antibacterial properties.

Immunological aspects of breast feeding

A number of defensive factors are present in breast milk, including (a) lysozyme, (b) lactoperoxidase, (c) lactoferrin (which sequestrates iron needed by pathogens), (d) immunoglobulins, especially IgA and complement, (e) antistaphylococcal factor and (f) neutrophils. In addition, breast milk promotes intestinal growth of *Lactobacillus bifidus,* which maintains a low intestinal pH and thereby inhibits growth of potentially harmful bacteria.

Immunology of haemolytic disease of the newborn

The commonest cause of haemolytic disease in newborns is rhesus incompatibility, but other red cell antigens may be involved. Maternal sensitisation results from transplacental passage of antigen (e.g. rhesus) positive cells from the fetus. Red cells are likely to pass into the maternal circulation after delivery, abortion or trauma. Only a proportion (about 20%) of mothers exposed to the rhesus antigen will be immune, of whom half will have detectable antibody levels in the puerperium and the remainder will develop antibodies during the next pregnancy. ABO incompatibility between mother and fetus has a protective effect, because the fetal red cells are coated with anti-ABO antibodies.

Maternal sensitisation results in production of IgG antibodies (especially

IgG_1 and IgG_3). The familiar antibodies which lead to ABO incompatibility and transfusion reactions are IgM. Occasionally mothers may produce IgG antibodies against the fetal ABO system, which cross the placenta and lead to haemolysis in the incompatible fetus.

There are five types of rhesus antigen, called C, D, E, c and e; all are expressions of a gene at a single locus. D causes the most severe haemolytic reactions, followed by c and E. By convention, rhesus-positive individuals have D antigen and rhesus-negative subjects (15% of the Caucasian population) lack it. Rhesus-positive individuals may be homozygous or (more commonly) heterozygous for D. Some individuals have a slightly altered D antigen (D^u) which may result in antibody formation.

There are many other antigens apart from the rhesus and ABO systems – Kell, Duffy, M and N being the most important. Anti-Lewis antibodies are frequently encountered but these are not haemolytic as the antigen is adsorbed from plasma and is not an intrinsic part of the red cell membrane.

Neonates do not have ABO antibodies; these appear later as a cross-reaction to ingested antigens.

Chapter 4

Endocrinology

Basic concepts in endocrinology

Feedback control. Reproductive function is controlled by steroids from the gonads. These are produced by specific cells in the ovary and testis, which respond to pituitary gonadotrophins – luteinising hormone (LH) and follicle stimulating hormone (FSH). As with many other hormones, sex steroids inhibit secretion of their trophic hormones (negative feedback). Under a specific set of circumstances, oestrogen may stimulate secretion of gonadotrophins (positive feedback).

Receptors. Protein hormones exert their effect on target cells by combining with cell surface receptors. Steroid receptors are located predominantly in the nucleus. The receptor is made up of one steroid binding unit and two non-binding subunits. The binding unit has one binding site for steroid and one for DNA; the latter attaches to short pelindromic sequences of DNA ('hormone responsive elements') upstream of the target genes. Receptor molecules which are not attached to steroid cannot bind with DNA because the DNA binding site is capped with a specific protein known as heat-shock protein 90 (HSP 90). The combination of steroid with receptor causes a conformational change, after which it can displace the HSP 90. All the nuclear steroid receptors are members of a single family of proteins. The receptors for thyroid hormone and retinoic acid are part of the same family. The binding units of these receptors are structurally related to some oncogenes. The biological activity is maintained only for as long as the receptor is occupied by the hormone. Thus steroids such as oestrogen, whose receptors have long half-lives, are present in lower concentrations than others, such as progesterone and cortisol, whose receptors have short half-lives.

Second messenger system. Larger protein hormones, such as the trophic hormones, cannot enter the cell. They combine with a surface receptor which activates adenyl cyclase in the cell membrane. This catalyses production of a second messenger, cyclic adenosine 3′,5′-monophosphate (cyclic AMP), from ATP. Excessive build-up of this substance is prevented by another enzyme, phosphodiesterase. Cyclic AMP activates protein kinases, which cause phosphorylation, and thereby activation of specific enzymes. A second and very similar system involves formation of inositol triphosphate. The surface receptor has three loops outside the cell, three loops in the cytoplasm and seven transmembrane domains. The extracellular domain is specific to the individual hormone, although LH and human chorionic gonadotrophin (hCG) act through the same receptor.

Biosynthesis of protein and peptide hormones.   Protein hormones are synthesised on ribosomes and stored by the Golgi apparatus in separate vesicles within the same cell. They are released into the circulation by fusion of these vesicles with the cell membrane, a process involving entry of calcium into the cell and contraction of myofibrils. Connections with neighbouring cells, through gap junctions, synchronise this process. Excess vesicles are phagocytosed by lysosomes. Most protein hormones are modified after they have been formed on the ribosomes. For example, ACTH and insulin are cleaved from larger molecules, and hCG, LH, FSH and thyroid-stimulating hormone (TSH) gain a carbohydrate moiety before they are secreted.

Protein binding of hormones.   All steroid hormones (and thyronines) are carried in blood largely bound to proteins. It is only the 'free' fraction that is able to move into cells and exert a biological effect. If there is an increase in binding proteins the free fraction is diminished; a compensatory increase in trophic hormone then occurs and restores the total amount of free hormone.

Hypothalamus

Functional anatomy

The functional anatomy of the hypothalamus and pituitary is shown in Fig. 4.1. The median eminence of the hypothalamus is connected to the pituitary gland by the pituitary stalk. The hypothalamus stretches from the optic chiasm in front to the mamillary bodies behind. The hypothalamus receives its arterial supply from the circle of Willis, and the supra-optic nucleus (see below) has the richest blood supply of any area in the brain. Capillaries draining the median eminence enter the portal system, which passes into the anterior pituitary.

Many nuclear groups – hypothalamic centres – exist in the hypothalamus. The paraventricular and supra-optic centres synthesise posterior pituitary hormones and the ventromedial nuclei control satiety, but specific functions cannot be attributed to the other centres in humans.

The median eminence contains terminals of many peptide-secreting neurons whose cell bodies are situated in the hypothalamic centres. These nerve terminals are closely applied to the looped capillaries in this region and contain the pituitary releasing and inhibiting hormones. The activity of the central nervous system is converted into chemical signals, and the hypothalamus,

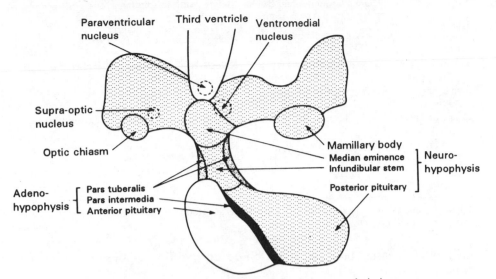

Fig. 4.1. Functional anatomy of the hypothalamus and pituitary.

together with the adrenal medulla and pineal gland, is referred to as a neuro-endocrine transducer.

In addition, the portal vessels in the median eminence are connected to the fluid of the third ventricle by specialised ciliated ependymal cells called tanycytes.

Hypothalamic control of the pituitary

Minute amounts of pituitary regulating hormones are released into the portal veins, leading to secretion of much greater amounts of pituitary hormones, and there is, in turn, a magnifying effect of the pituitary hormones on the target gland. The secretion of hypothalamic peptides is regulated by 'higher' neural centres and also by a negative feedback mechanism whereby target gland hormones alter secretion of hypothalamic hormones or interfere with their action at the pituitary level. Generally, both the hypothalamic and pituitary sites are important, but in thyroid and gonadal function control is exerted mainly through pituitary feedback.

The hypothalamic pituitary regulating substances (Table 4.1) stimulate both secretion and synthesis of pituitary hormones. Injection of a releasing hormone results in a rapid rise in the trophic hormone, reaching a maximum level after about 20 min. The greater the secretion of endogenous releasing hormone, the greater is the response to an exogenous releasing factor. Thus in thyrotoxicosis the response to thyrotrophin-releasing hormone (TRH) is less than normal, whereas in primary hypothyroidism it is greater. Similarly, in the prepubertal state there is little gonadotrophin response to gonadotrophin-releasing hormone (GnRH) as basal secretion of releasing hormone is very low. After the menopause, when negative feedback by the ovary is reduced,

Table 4.1. Hypothalamic hormones and factors affecting anterior pituitary cells

Hormones	*Effect on anterior pituitary*
Gonadotrophin-releasing hormone (GnRH) (decapeptide)	Release of LH and FSH
Thyrotrophin-releasing hormone (TRH) (Tripeptide)	Release of thyroid-stimulating hormone and prolactin[a]
Somatostatin (growth hormone-inhibiting hormone) (14 amino acids)	Inhibition of growth hormone
Corticotrophin-releasing hormone (CRH) (42 amino acids)	Release of adrenocorticotrophic hormone (ACTH)
Growth hormone-releasing hormone (40 amino acids)	Release of growth hormone
Factor	
Prolactin-inhibiting factor (dopamine)	Inhibition of prolactin and growth hormone

[a] Under some circumstances additional factors are affected, e.g. TRH causes an increase of ACTH during pregnancy

high basal releasing hormone secretion occurs and the response to GnRH is enhanced.

GnRH stimulates secretion of both LH and FSH. The fact that LH and FSH diverge during the menstrual cycle, i.e. that one level may fall while the other stays the same, is ascribed to a modifying action of gonadal steroids on pituitary gonadotrophin-releasing cells. Thus increasing levels of oestrogen cause proportionately more LH to be released than FSH in response to a given amount of GnRH.

Before puberty the gonads and secondary sexual tissues are capable of response to appropriate hormonal stimuli, and the ovary at birth may contain advanced (tertiary) follicles owing to stimulation by hCG. Similarly, female babies may have a vaginal bleed 2 or 3 days after birth due to 'menstrual' shedding of the endometrium as a result of withdrawal of their high oestrogen environment. As puberty approaches, there is an FSH response to GnRH; later, as gonadal steroid levels increase, LH secretion also occurs and eventually exceeds that of FSH.

Many releasing/inhibiting substances are found in sites outside the pituitary. The most ubiquitous is somatostatin, which is found in D cells of pancreatic islets (where it inhibits gastrin), the stomach (where it inhibits acid and pepsin secretion) and the small intestine (where it inhibits secretion of cholecystokinin, vaso-active intestinal peptide and motilin). Local modulating action of this nature is referred to as a paracrine effect.

The hypothalamus secretes releasing hormones as a series of pulses, and the release is determined by the frequency rather than the amplitude of these pulses. All anterior pituitary hormones are secreted in pulses lasting less than 90 min. Continuous administration of releasing hormone may, paradoxically, inhibit secretion of the relevant trophic hormone. Thus sustained release of implants of GnRH is antigonadotrophic and contraceptive. The phenomenon is ascribed to down-regulation of the pituitary receptor due to endocytosis of the hormone–receptor complex. A number of neurotransmitters within the hypothalamus regulate the secretion of releasing factors and hormones. These include dopamine, noradrenaline, calcitonin, γ-aminobutyric acid, serotonin, substance P and endorphins. Endorphins have the following effects: (a) a decrease in dopamine secretion, thereby increasing prolactin secretion; (b) an increase in growth hormone secretion; and (c) a decrease in gonadotrophin secretion due to a decrease in the frequency of GnRH pulses.

The output of ACTH, growth hormone and prolactin varies with the time of day and this is regulated by the hypothalamus. ACTH output is highest between 6 a.m. and 9 a.m. Similarly, the hypothalamus is responsible for greater TSH secretion in cold climates. In addition, the hypothalamus is concerned with autonomic reflexes controlling body temperature and with the regulation of caloric balance.

Anterior pituitary

Anatomy and embryology

The anterior pituitary forms from Rathke's pouch, an upward evagination of the ectoderm of the pharyngeal roof. From the upper part cells proliferate to form the pars tuberalis, which partly encircles the pituitary stalk; the posterior part forms the pars intermedia, which is prominent in the fetus but becomes atrophic at birth.

The pituitary lies in a depression in the sphenoid, the sella turcica. The sella turcica is covered by a layer of dura mater (the diaphragma sellae) through which the pituitary stalk passes.

Immediately above the pituitary gland lies the hypothalamus and in front of this is the optic chiasm. Laterally and above lie the cavernous sinuses and oculomotor nerves. The pituitary is supplied with blood by the portal system originating in the hypothalamus (80%) and by a direct arterial supply. The internal carotid gives rise to a superior pituitary artery (which supplies the stalk and, via the 'artery of the tubercula', the posterior pituitary) and an inferior pituitary artery.

The pituitary increases in weight by 30%–50% during pregnancy due to an increase in prolactin-secreting cells.

Micro-anatomy

The anterior pituitary cells are surrounded by a rich network of capillary sinusoids. On light microscopy the cells can be divided by their staining reaction with haematoxylin and eosin into acidophils, basophils and chromophobes, which represent sparsely granulated eosinophils or basophils. Acidophils secrete prolactin and growth hormone, and the basophilic cells secrete TSH, LH, FSH and pro-opiomelanocortin. Acidophils are situated mostly in the posterolateral part of the gland and undergo hyperplasia in pregnancy.

Growth hormone, ACTH and TSH

Growth Hormone (GH) is a protein with no carbohydrate residues and a molecular weight of 21 500; the chemical structure is similar to that of human placental lactogen (hPL) and prolactin. As with the latter, it is coded on chromosome 17. In the circulation it is associated with a binding protein, which is identical to the extracellular domain of the membrane GH receptor. It is responsible for growth in children (but not in the fetus) and, with other factors, for the control of carbohydrate and lipid metabolism. It is secreted in short bursts, most of which occur in the first part of the night. These bursts are more frequent in children. Secretion is also stimulated by stress, hypoglycaemia and certain amino acids (especially arginine) and is inhibited by glucose and corticosteroids. The main metabolic effects are stimulation of lipolysis and insulin antagonism. The growth-promoting effects are mediated at the tissue level through insulin-like growth factors (IGFs) of molecular weight circa 7000.

Pygmies have normal levels of GH but low levels of IGF-1. IGF levels are lower in the fetus than in the adult. GH secretion is reduced during pregnancy.

Adrenocorticotrophic hormone is a polypeptide of molecular weight 4500 containing 39 amino acids. The first 24 are responsible for the biological effects. The first 13 are identical to α-MSH (melanocyte-stimulating hormone), and amino acids 18–39 correspond to CLIP (corticotrophin-like intermediate lobe peptide). These two peptides are secreted by the intermediate lobe in fetal life but are not present in blood during postnatal life. ACTH has some pigmentary activity and this accounts for the skin changes in Addison's disease. ACTH-secreting cells also make a 91-amino-acid substance (β-lipotrophin, β-LPH), whose function is unknown. Within the sequence of β-LPH lies the amino acid sequence of two brain peptides that have opiate-like effects: β-endorphin (residues 61–91) and met-enkephalin (61–65).

All of these molecules are derived from three families of opioid peptides, each derived from a precursor: the β-endorphin/ACTH precursor (pro-opiomelanocortin, POMC); the enkephalin precursor (pro-enkephalin or pro-enkephalin A); and the dynorphin/neo-endorphin precursor (pro-dynorphin or pro-enkephalin B).

Circulating ACTH levels increase during pregnancy, as do levels of total and unbound cortisol.

Thyroid-stimulating hormone is a glycoprotein. It is composed of two peptide chains (α and β) and has a similar structure to other glycoprotein hormones, LH, FSH and hCG. The α-subunits are almost identical in all these compounds and biological specificity resides in the β-subunits (although the two subunits must be combined for biological activity).

Gonadotrophins and prolactin

Gonadotrophins (LH and FSH)

Chemical composition.   As with TSH and hCG, LH and FSH are glycoproteins composed of two subunits, α and β.

The gonadotrophins have molecular weights of around 28 000. They are metabolised in the liver and kidneys and a significant fraction is excreted in urine. LH has a half-life of around 20 min and FSH about twice this.

Pattern of gonadotrophin secretion in the menstrual cycle (Fig. 4.2).   For most of the cycle, gonadotrophins are controlled by a negative feedback of oestrogen (and, to a lesser extent, of progesterone). LH and FSH are therefore at their lowest levels during the luteal phase of the cycle, when steroid levels are highest. Their levels tend to rise during menstruation as steroid levels fall. During the follicular phase, FSH levels are suppressed but LH levels remain steady. Shortly before ovulation there is a surge of LH with a simultaneous smaller FSH rise. This is due to *positive* feedback from the relatively high oestrogen levels in the late follicular phase.

Control of gonadotrophin secretion.   Significant secretion occurs only in the presence of GnRH, which is secreted in hypothalamic nuclei, particularly by the arcuate nucleus, and released into the portal system from the median eminence. Direct feedback by oestrogen is another important controlling factor. Oestrogens exert both negative and positive feedback and also alter the proportion of LH and FSH secreted in response to a given amount of GnRH: higher concentrations of oestrogens cause proportionately more LH to be released. Thus the low-oestrogen status before the menarche and after the menopause is characterised by relatively greater concentrations of FSH. Similarly, as the follicular phase progresses, the increasing oestrogen levels bring about a continuously increasing LH:FSH ratio (see Fig. 4.2).

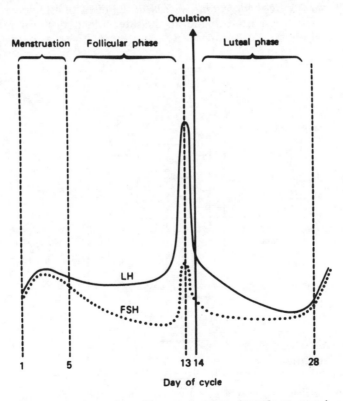

Fig. 4.2.   The pattern of gonadotrophin secretion throughout the menstrual cycle.

Oestrogen feedback is mediated mainly through the pituitary rather than the hypothalamus; the LH surge and ovulation can take place in the presence of a constant amount of GnRH.

Gonadotrophin-releasing hormone is released in pulses. Very frequent pulses or continuous administration cause a diminished gonadotrophin response because of depletion (down-regulation) of the receptor for GnRH. Less frequent pulses (once every 3 h) cause no change in LH but an increase in FSH, a pattern which characterises early puberty. Pulses of very large amplitude cause relatively more LH to be secreted. There is no increase in the GnRH pulse frequency during the mid-cycle gonadotrophin surge.

Secretion of GnRH is influenced by negative (and sometimes positive) feedback effects of oestrogen, and negative feedback by progesterone and testosterone. The effects of these target organ hormones on the hypothalamus are referred to as long feedback loops to distinguish them from short feedback loops whereby gonadotrophins cause a suppressive effect on GnRH secretion (ultra-short feedback applies to a possible suppressive effect of GnRH on itself). Prolactin also diminishes GnRH secretion, as do many pineal hormones and emotional factors such as stress. These interrelationships are shown in Fig. 4.3. The effects on GnRH secretion are probably mediated via neurotransmitters such as noradrenaline, dopamine and endorphin.

General patterns of gonadotrophin secretion.   Pulses of LH secretion occur every 1–2 h. The frequency is higher in the later follicular phase and lower in the mid-luteal phase. The mid-cycle LH surge usually starts between 5 a.m.

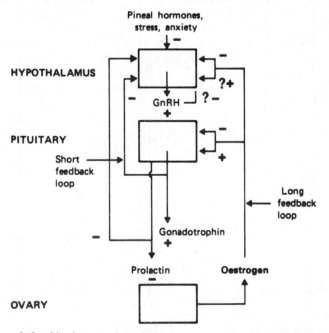

Fig. 4.3.   Interrelationships between hypothalamus, pituitary and ovary. In males, testosterone exerts negative feedback at both pituitary and hypothalamic levels.

and 9 a.m. The surge is biphasic, lasting a total of 30 h. The initial rapid rise occurs over about 12 h and is sometimes accompanied by a slight drop in temperature. Ovulation occurs 36–38 h after the start of the LH surge, and 16–26 h after the LH peak.

Gonadotrophins in the fetus. Gonadotrophins reach a peak at about 20 weeks of intrauterine life and another peak in the first 1–2 months of infancy (Fig. 4.4). In the male, levels of LH and testosterone are evaluated for the first 3–6 months of life.

In the male fetus high levels of testosterone are secreted under the influence of hCG and maintained by pituitary gonadotrophins. In the female the maximum rate of oogenesis occurs at the peak of gonadotrophin secretion. During fetal life gonadotrophin levels are higher in the female fetus, whereas in the male they are suppressed by the elevated testosterone levels. The increase in FSH after birth is also greater in female infants.

Prolactin

Chemical composition. Prolactin is chemically similar to growth hormone; it is a protein with a molecular weight of 24 000. There are also large polymeric forms ('big' prolactin). A glycosylated form of prolactin is secreted by the endometrium in the luteal phase of the cycle, and by the decidua in pregnancy.

Control of secretion. Prolactin is the only pituitary hormone which is inhibited rather than stimulated by hypothalamic factors. The main prolactin inhibitory factor is dopamine, and drugs that are dopamine antagonists (e.g. phenothiazines and metoclopramide) potentiate prolactin release. Serotonin and TRH stimulate prolactin release, and oestrogen causes increased prolactin synthesis. The number of prolactin-secreting cells increases dramatically during pregnancy. The half-life is 5–10 min.

Action of prolactin. High levels inhibit pulsatile GnRH secretion and

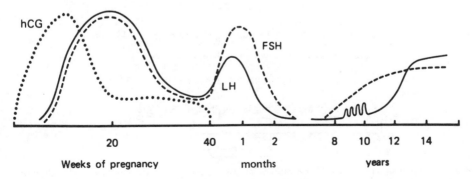

Fig. 4.4. Gonadotrophin levels throughout life.

oestrogen secretion by the ovary. In many animals, but not in humans, prolactin is essential for corpus luteum function.

Pattern of prolactin secretion.   High levels in the fetus decline rapidly after birth. Levels are higher in girls than in boys after puberty and are slightly higher in the luteal part of the cycle. Levels increase steadily during pregnancy, reaching values 10–20 times those in the non-pregnant state. In the absence of suckling, levels return to normal 2–3 weeks after delivery. There is a long-term decrease in the non-pregnancy levels of prolactin in women who have had many pregnancies. There is a circadian variation, with high levels in the first part of the night. At all times the pattern of release is pulsatile.

Posterior pituitary

The posterior pituitary (neurohypophysis) is a neurosecretory gland. The cell bodies lie in the hypothalamus, and the axon and axon terminals make up the stalk and the gland itself. The axon terminals are closely associated with capillaries as a neurohaemal organ. The hormones are the nonapeptides (nine amino acids) oxytocin and vasopressin (Fig. 4.5). Both peptides are secreted by the supra-optic and paraventricular nuclei of the hypothalamus, although vasopressin predominates in the supra-optic nucleus. The hormones are transported as granules down the nerve axons and stored in the axon terminals prior to release. The granules contain the active hormone and carrier proteins (neurophysin), both of which arise from the same large precursor molecule.

The main physiological action of arginine-vasopressin (antidiuretic hormone) is to increase the permeability of the renal collecting system to water; in the absence of vasopressin there is an inability to concentrate the urine (diabetes insipidus). Secretion is controlled by the osmotic pressure of extracellular fluids via osmoreceptors in the hypothalamus. It is stimulated by nicotine and inhibited by alcohol. The pressor effect of vasopressin is of

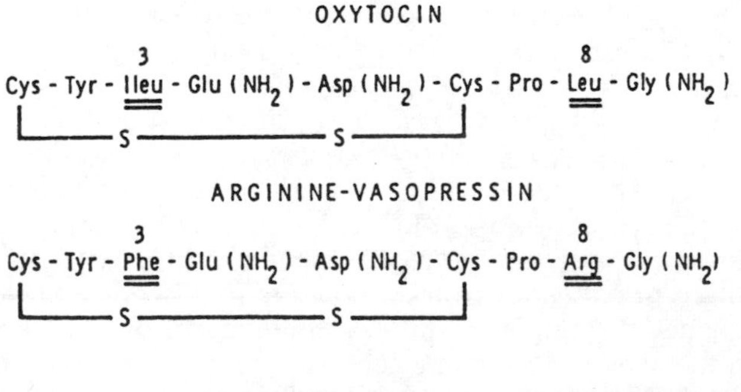

OXYTOCIN

$$Cys - Tyr - \underset{3}{Ileu} - Glu\,(NH_2) - Asp\,(NH_2) - Cys - Pro - \underset{8}{Leu} - Gly\,(NH_2)$$

ARGININE-VASOPRESSIN

$$Cys - Tyr - \underset{3}{Phe} - Glu\,(NH_2) - Asp\,(NH_2) - Cys - Pro - \underset{8}{Arg} - Gly\,(NH_2)$$

Fig. 4.5. The structures of oxytocin and arginine-vasopressin. Humans make arginine-vasopressin, whereas some animals, such as the pig, secrete lysine-vasopressin.

no significance under normal circumstances, but substantial elevations may be seen in acute events such as haemorrhage and anoxia.

Oxytocin has two main actions: (a) stimulation of the uterus, and (b) stimulation of the myoepithelial cells of the breast to cause milk ejection. In human pregnancy maternal oxytocin is released in spurts during the active and expulsive phases of labour, probably as the result of a neural reflex originating in the cervix and lower genital tract (Ferguson's reflex). Oxytocin (and vasopressin) is also released by the fetal pituitary during labour. The maternal circulation contains a placental enzyme, oxytocinase, which can split oxytocin, although this action is not thought to be of any physiological significance. During suckling there is a spurt release of oxytocin as the result of a reflex from nerve endings in the nipple. In the male there is release of oxytocin during orgasm.

Breast and lactation

Anatomy

The mature breast consists of glandular tissue, fibrous tissue joining the lobes and fat between the lobes. Fibrous strands (suspensory ligaments of Cooper) extend from the fibrous tissue to the overlying skin. There are 15–20 lobes, each consisting of 20–40 lobules which in turn include 10–100 alveoli. The ducts unite to form a single duct draining each lobe. They converge towards the areola, beneath which each duct has a dilatation, the lactiferous sinus. The areola contains numerous sebaceous glands (Montgomery) which become prominent in pregnancy and secrete a bactericidal lubricant.

The blood supply is from thoracic branches of the axillary artery and from the internal thoracic and intercostal arteries. The nerve supply is from cutaneous branches of the 4th, 5th and 6th thoracic nerves. Lymphatics from the central and lateral part of the breast drain into the axillary glands while those from the medial part drain into the mammary nodes, the subdiaphragmatic nodes and across the midline to the opposite axilla.

Development of the breast

The breast is an ectodermal structure. In the early fetus (6–7 weeks of embryonic life) a mammary gland (milk line) appears on either side of the midline; in humans the cephalic end of this thickens to form mammary buds. Each bud sprouts 15–20 epithelial cords, which at 20 weeks become canalised. Further proliferation and branching continues up to term, but in the neonate the breast becomes quiescent and no further changes occur until puberty.

At puberty there is a further proliferation of ducts and lobular organisation appears. However, true alveoli only appear during pregnancy. In early pregnancy there is extensive proliferation and lobulo-alveolar development; in later pregnancy the emphasis shifts to cell hypertrophy and appearance of secretions in the alveoli. Branching continues up to term and a small amount of colostrum may be secreted in the neonate. Overall the weight of the breast increases two- to three-fold and the blood-flow doubles.

Histology of the lactating mammary gland

The alveolar epithelium consists of short columnar cells with a microvillous surface. There is a prominent endoplasmic reticulum and Golgi apparatus at the base of the cell; fat droplets form at the apex. Both fat droplets and vesicles from the Golgi apparatus (protein and lactose) fuse with the cell membrane and are discharged into the lumen. Milk is stored in the alveoli, ducts and cisterns.

When lactation ceases there is extensive degeneration of lactogenic cells, a phagocytic reaction and fatty infiltration.

Hormonal control of breast growth and lactation

Breast growth during pregnancy is associated with increased levels of a complex of hormones including oestrogens, progesterone, hPL and prolactin from the maternal pituitary. Oestrogens promote duct growth, while alveolar development depends on the full complex of hormones. Progesterone inhibits the lactogenic (milk secretion) effects of hPL and prolactin. Although secretion of prolactin decreases by 50% after delivery, the rapidly decreasing levels of progesterone permit the full lactogenic action of residual prolactin, and milk secretion begins. In the absence of suckling, maternal levels of prolactin subsequently decrease slowly to reach non-pregnant values after 2–3 weeks. The suckling stimulus leads to sharp peaks of prolactin secretion and elevated basal levels, but this response diminishes progressively over 3 months of breastfeeding. There appears, therefore, to be little or no direct relationship between prolactin levels and milk yield. The most important controlling factor is regular removal of milk from the breast, which in turn promotes further milk secretion. In the absence of breastfeeding, prolactin levels return to normal 4 weeks postpartum and first menses occurs around 9 weeks. Because of a lack of pulsatile LH secretion the early cycles are often anovular. In women who breastfeed menstruation resumes in 28 weeks on average.

Milk ejection (release of preformed milk, not rapid secretion) is brought about by the contraction of myoepithelial cells around the alveoli and ducts under the influence of pituitary oxytocin. Oxytocin is released as a result of a neural reflex (the milk ejection reflex) originating from the suckling stimulus to the nipple. Suckling also inhibits the GnRH pulse generator, probably the main mechanism responsible for anovulation during breastfeeding.

Composition of milk

For 2–4 days after delivery the breast secretion is colostrum, a yellow fluid containing fat-laden cells (colostral corpuscles) and large quantities of protein and minerals. Colostrum and early breast milk contain relatively high levels of IgG, IgM and IgA, including antibodies to a variety of organisms, especially *E. coli*. After the first week the predominant immunoglobulin is secretory IgA.

The composition of human breast milk and a comparison with cow's milk are shown in Table 4.2.

Table 4.2. Composition of human breast and cow's milk

Component	Human	Cow
Protein[a]	1%–1.5% (40% casein)	3.3% (80% casein)
Carbohydrate[b]	7%	4.5%
Fat[c]	4%	4%
Minerals	0.2%	0.75%
Vitamins A, B, C, D[d]		
Growth factors		

[a] Lactalbumin, lactoglobulins, lactoferrin, casein.
[b] Mainly lactose, synthesised by the mammary epithelial cell from glucose and galactose.
[c] Triglycerides (olein, palmitin, stearin). Human milk contains relatively more olein and cow's milk more fatty acids (butyric acid, capric acid).
[d] Vitamin A is abundant; vitamins C and D may be deficient.

Sex steroids

Steroid hormones are based on a nucleus of three six-carbon rings (A, B and C) and one five-carbon ring (the D ring).

Steroid hormones are divided into three classes based on the number of carbon atoms: C-21 (e.g. progesterone, cortisol, aldosterone), C-19 (e.g. testosterone and androstenedione) and C-18 (oestrogens).

Biosynthesis

The biosynthetic pathways for all steroid-producing glands are shown in Fig. 4.6. All steroid-producing organs, with the exception of the placenta, can synthesise cholesterol from acetate. However, most cholesterol is derived from blood, and in particular that fraction bound to low density lipoprotein (LDL); there are specific LDL receptors on the cells. During the subsequent steps of steroid synthesis carbon atoms can only be reduced, never increased. Specific enzymes determine which steroid is produced by a particular cell. The conversion of cholesterol to pregnenolone is an adenyl cyclase-dependent process in the mitochondria and is the rate-limiting step of steroidogenesis. This is the level at which trophic hormones, such as LH, exert their effect. Most of the subsequent conversions take place in the microsomes of the endoplasmic reticulum.

There is evidence for pulsatile release of sex steroids, but the pulses are not always coincident with those of gonadotrophins.

Urinary excretion

Steroids can only be excreted in urine after conjugation with other molecules (glucuronides and sulphates), which render them soluble in water. This process eliminates most of the biological activity. There is a delay of up to 48 h between the peak level of a steroid in blood and the peak of the conjugate in urine.

Oestrogens

In the premenopausal female ovarian oestradiol is the major oestrogen. Oestrogens are also formed in peripheral tissues, particularly skin and fat, by conversion of androstenedione. This is an important source of oestrogen in the male (50%) and in the postmenopausal female. Tissues that react to oestrogens have a specific intranuclear receptor protein. Oestrogens bind

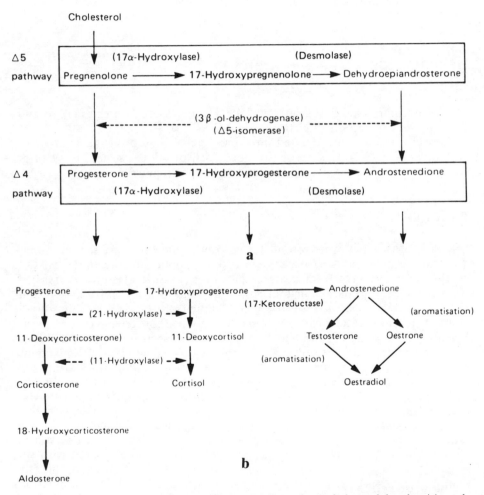

Fig. 4.6. **a** Synthesis of the key steroid intermediates from cholesterol by the Δ4- and Δ5-pathways. **b** Synthesis of the major steroid groups (glucocorticoids, mineralocorticoids and sex steroids) from the intermediates shown in **a**. **c** Structures of some of the principal steroids in **a** and **b**.

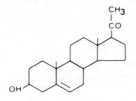

Pregnenolone

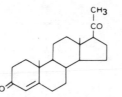

Progesterone

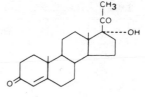

17-Hydroxyprogesterone

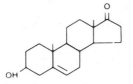

Dehydroepiandrosterone

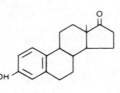

Androstenedione

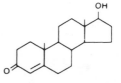

Testosterone

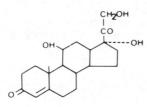

Cortisol

Oestrone

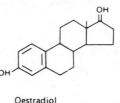

Oestradiol

Fig. 4.6c

to this protein; the complex binds to and activates DNA. Among proteins produced in this way is the progesterone receptor. Thus the effects of progesterone are dependent on oestrogen 'priming'. Stronger oestrogens, such as oestradiol, bind more avidly to the receptor than weaker oestrogens such as oestriol. Anti-oestrogenic agents such as progestagens and clomiphene deplete the oestrogen receptor. The actions of oestrogens are summarised in Table 4.3.

All steroids bind to albumin and in addition there are specific binding proteins in plasma. Oestradiol (E_2) and testosterone bind to the same binding protein, sex hormone-binding globulin (SHBG). This is a high-affinity low-capacity β-glycoprotein synthesised by the liver (albumin has a low affinity but high capacity). SHBG binds approximately 80% of E_2 in blood. Nineteen per cent of E_2 is bound to albumin, and 1% is free and biologically active. Oestriol (E_3) is not bound to SHBG; 30% is bound to albumin.

Metabolism of oestrogens takes place principally in the liver. The steroid molecules are conjugated with glucuronide (and to a small extent with sulphate) to form water-soluble products, which are excreted in urine or bile (the major route). A small proportion of E_2 is converted to E_3 prior to conjugation. Deconjugation by intestinal bacteria leads to reabsorption (enterohepatic circulation). The half-life of circulating oestrogens is 5–25 min.

Additionally, small amounts of oestrogens are metabolised by hydroxylation

Table 4.3. Actions of oestrogens

1. Secondary sexual characteristics	Growth of vulva Development of the breasts and female distribution of fat Hypertrophy of vaginal wall. Increased glycogen content and resulting decrease in pH. Increased number of cells in epithelium; large mature surface cells with small nuclei Growth of body of uterus Fusion of epiphyses (increase in bone age) Changes in shape of bony pelvis
2. Menstruation functions	Negative and positive feedback on pituitary and hypothalamus Proliferative phase of endometrium Together with progesterone promote secretory changes
3. Maturation of the oocyte	Dependent on high blood concentrations of oestrogen
4. Physiological and anatomical changes in pregnancy	Breast development Hypertrophy and hyperplasia of the myometrium and increased excitability of uterus (an effect counteracted by progesterone)
5. Metabolic effects	Calcification of bone Possible increase in renin and angiotensin Diminished peripheral glucose uptake Increased thyroxine, cortisol and sex hormone-binding globulin Increase in cholesterol and triglycerides Decrease in high-density lipoproteins Increase in factors VII, VIII, IX and X Decrease in fibrinolysis Inhibition of conversion of tryptophan to serotonin Decrease in blood and urine calcium

at the 2 and 4 positions to yield catecholoestrogens. The latter will bind to oestrogen receptors but will not activate them and are therefore anti-oestrogens. Catecholoestrogens can also inhibit breakdown of catecholamines, bind to pituitary dopamine receptors, and induce LH release. They may play an important part in the control of pituitary function.

Progesterone

Progesterone is derived from the ovary but with a small adrenal contribution. The daily production increases ten-fold during the luteal phase to reach 20–30 mg/day.

Progesterone depends on the presence of oestrogen in order to exert its biological effects. These include:

1. *Vagina*: large superficial cells with small pyknotic nuclei are replaced by small cells with large nuclei

2. *Cervical mucus*: becomes thicker, opaque and less abundant

3. *Endometrium*: secretory changes

4. *Uterus*: the threshold for uterine excitation increases, resulting in low-frequency high-amplitude contractions

5. *Other smooth muscle*: general relaxant effect

6. *Breast*: glandular development

7. *Metabolic effects*: progesterone is thermogenic, opposes the sodium-retaining effects of aldosterone, increases the respiratory minute volume (and thereby reduces alveolar and blood P_{CO_2}) and has catabolic effects resulting in increased urinary nitrogen excretion

The intracellular progesterone receptor (induced by the action of oestrogen) acts similarly to the oestrogen receptor. Seventy per cent of circulating progesterone is bound to cortisol-binding globulin.

Progesterone is metabolised to a variety of products, including pregnanediol. These metabolites are converted by the liver to water-soluble glucuronides or sulphates. About 20% of progesterone is excreted as pregnanediol glucuronide.

Testosterone

Testosterone is produced by the Leydig cells of the testis, and male levels are 10 times higher than female. In the male there is a transient increase in testosterone in the first week of neonatal life, and another increase at 2–3 months. The source of androgens in women is shown in Table 4.4.

In the male, testosterone is responsible for development of the wolffian duct and external genitalia (it is *not* responsible for involution of the müllerian system). It is also responsible for secondary sexual development at puberty and for spermatogenesis, and may play a small part in development of male psychology. In the normal female its role is less clear, but, together with androstenedione, it is responsible for the development of pubic and axillary hair. The former is one of the first signs of puberty.

Sectoli cell → MIS

Table 4.4. The source of various androgenic steroids and their precursors in the circulation of women (see also Figs. 4.6, 4.7)

Steroid	Ovary (%)	Adrenal (%)	Peripheral conversion (%)	Secretion rate (mg/day)
Testosterone	20	30	50[a]	0.2
Androstenedione	30	60	10[b]	2.5
Dehydroepiandrosterone (and DHEASO$_4$)		80		10
Dihydrotestosterone			100[c]	

[a] Of ovarian and adrenal androstenedione.
[b] Of dehydroepiandrosterone.
[c] Only 15% from testosterone, remainder from androstenedione and DHEA; note that plasma DHT probably does *not* reflect intracellular DHT.

Table 4.5. Binding of testosterone to plasma proteins

	Male (%)	Female (%)
'Free'	2	1
Albumin-bound	38	19
SHBG-bound	60	80

Androgens exert their effect by binding to an intracellular receptor. In most tissues testosterone itself binds very weakly to the receptor and must first be converted to dihydrotestosterone (DHT) by the enzyme 5α-reductase; DHT is 100 times more potent than the parent compound. This conversion is essential in hair follicles and in the development of the urogenital sinus and urogenital tubercle into the male external genitalia and prostate. The effects of testosterone on muscle, the wolffian duct and the central nervous system occur without any prior conversion.

The carrier proteins for testosterone are sex hormone-binding globulin (SHBG) and albumin; the binding constant of SHBG for testosterone is 3 times that of E_2. Because of the higher concentrations of SHBG and the lower concentration of testosterone in the female, only 1% of testosterone is free (compared with 2% in the male). Table 4.5 summarises the binding of testosterone to plasma proteins.

SHBG levels are depressed by testosterone and increased by oestradiol. Levels are therefore highest in females during pregnancy and lowest in males after puberty. Synthesis of SHBG is stimulated by oestrogens and thyroxine, and inhibited by insulin, growth hormone, androgenic drugs and progestagens. Concentrations are lower in obese subjects.

Androgens are partly metabolised to androsterone and aetiocholanolone prior to excretion in urine as the water-soluble sulphate or glucuronide. Dehydroepiandrosterone is excreted almost entirely as the glucuronide. The principal 18-oxosteroids, androsterone and aetiocholanolone, occur predominantly as the glucuronides with about 10% as sulphates. Dihydrotestosterone is excreted as 3α- and 3β-androstenediols.

Ovary

Development of primordial follicles

Numerous primordial follicles consisting of a primary oocyte and a single layer of spindle-shaped granulosa cells are scattered throughout the ovarian stroma. The granulosa cells become cuboidal and proliferate to form the multilayered primary follicles.

Some 3 months before ovulation, about 300 follicles are recruited for development. Only 30 of these become gonadotrophin dependent and will commence rapid growth at the beginning of the menstrual cycle. Small numbers are also formed during late fetal life and childhood and tend to push the primordial follicles into the peripheral cortex. Secondary follicles are characterised by the formation of a large fluid-filled cavity – the antrum.

This is accomplished through coalescence of many small cavities which appear among the granulosa cells; these small cavities with their surrounding rosette of granulosa cells are called Call–Exner bodies. The fluid, liquor folliculi, is formed by transudation and secretion from surrounding cells.

The granulosa cells project into the antrum in the area of the primary oocyte, forming a mound known as the cumulus oophorus. A homogeneous layer, the zona pellucida, is secreted around the oocyte by the granulosa cells, which nevertheless maintain contact by means of thin cytoplasmic processes (gap junctions) that penetrate this layer. The surrounding ovarian stroma cells form a compact layer, the theca interna, which is separated from the granulosa cells by a basement membrane. A loose layer of stroma cells, the theca externa, envelops the whole structure.

Only one or two follicles undergo further development in any cycle. This involves the rapid expansion of the antrum and thinning out of the follicle wall within 48 h of ovulation to form the tertiary follicle. Fully grown follicles are 2–3 cm in diameter.

Extensive changes occur on the cell surface of granulosa cells during the follicular cycle. Multiple microvilli containing microfilaments develop and are believed to carry the rapidly increasing numbers of gonadotrophin receptors, which amplify the follicular response in the preovulatory period. These microvilli are withdrawn in the luteal phase. The cytoplasm of granulosa cells is also the site of considerable changes; the smooth endoplasmic reticulum and mitochondria increase in preovulatory follicles. Central granulosa cells in the cumulus oophorus secrete glycosaminoglycans, while peripheral cells, near the basement membrane, synthesise plasminogen activator. Peripheral cells have more LH receptors and a greater number of gap junctions.

Further development of the oocyte

The primary oocyte enlarges from 35 to 100 μm diameter early in follicular development and undergoes no subsequent enlargement.

The nucleus is displaced to the periphery of the expanding cytoplasm. Peripheral cortical granules are formed from the Golgi apparatus; these contain the substances that will block polyspermic fertilisation. Energy is provided by the direct metabolism of pyruvate provided by cumulus cells; the mitochondria where this occurs are found in greatest concentration around a lamellar paranuclear structure called Babiani's vitelline body.

The first meiotic division begins during late fetal life but the process is interrupted at the diplotene stage until it is resumed 36 h before ovulation. One of the two daughter cells is small and is extruded as the first polar body. The secondary oocyte immediately enters the second meiotic division and remains in metaphase until fertilisation. Division is then completed, a second polar body extruded and the female pronucleus formed. The very prolonged meiosis of the primary oocyte is probably due to an inhibitory effect of the granulosa cells through their cytoplasmic extensions, and these are withdrawn before meiosis is resumed. During follicular maturation, granulosa cells deliver another substance, called male pronucleus growth factor, to the ovum. Thus ova separated from early follicles resume meiosis and may be fertilised but the pronucleus does not form adequately.

Corpus luteum

The corpus luteum is formed immediately after ovulation as a result of the following changes:

1. The follicle collapses after extrusion of the ovum and fluid and the central cavity fills with blood and fibrin.

2. The basement membrane separating the granulosa from the theca disappears and thecal capillaries enter the granulosa.

3. The cytoplasm of the granulosa and theca cells hypertrophies, with accumulation of lipid droplets and proliferation of the smooth endoplasmic reticulum and mitochondria (granulosa lutein and theca lutein cells).

4. Degeneration and formation of a corpus albicans begins after 10 days unless a pregnancy occurs.

Luteinisation of human follicles may sometimes occur without extrusion of the ovum. Progesterone production increases rapidly after extrusion of the ovum, although it begins to rise shortly before ovulation. Oestrogen production, which declines about 20 h before ovulation, recovers within a day. Both hormones peak after 6–8 days.

Corpus luteum function requires gonadotrophin support, notably from LH and to a much lesser extent from FSH. The number of LH receptors reaches a maximum during the mid-luteal phase. The corpus luteum can be sustained artificially by injections of hCG for at least 21 days beyond the expected time of the period. In a non-conceptual cycle luteolysis is probably programmed to occur at the cellular level and is initiated automatically at the time of ovulation.

Luteolysis begins with shunting of blood away from the corpus luteum, following which lysosomes initiate a process of lipolysis. A specific luteolytic factor has not been isolated in primates, but $PGF_{2\alpha}$ from the endometrium may fulfil this function in other species.

Steroid production by the ovary

Oestradiol is produced by the developing follicles; the dominant follicle (>10 mm diameter) secretes 90% of the total. The thecal cells, under the influence of LH, secrete androgenic precursors by the Δ5-pathway (Fig. 4.6a). FSH stimulates proliferation of granulosa cells, which acquire LH receptors and the enzyme aromatase cytochrome P450 (which is crucial for follicular oestrogen synthesis). In the late follicular phase follicle growth and oestrogen synthesis continue in response to LH and FSH jointly. Production of progesterone from pregnenolone does not begin until until the Δ4-pathway (Fig. 4.6a) is activated at ovulation. An increase occurs 24–48 h before ovulation (6 h after the start of the LH surge). The main postovulatory surge corresponds to luteinisation and vascularisation and reaches a peak 7–8 days after the LH peak. Small luteal cells (corresponding to theca) secrete progesterone and androgens under the influence of LH; large luteal cells (corresponding to granulosa) secrete oestrogens under the influence of FSH. Adrenal androgens (DHEA and $DHEASO_4$) show no change during the cycle.

Peptide hormone production by the ovary

The ovary produces a number of peptide hormones:

1. Oxytocin and vasopressin (in the corpus luteum of animals but not the human).

2. Relaxin: an insulin-like peptide produced by the corpus luteum of pregnancy. It augments softening of the connective tissue of the cervix and of the pelvic ligaments. Blood levels of relaxin reach a peak in the first trimester.

3. Inhibin: a protein of molecular weight 32 000 which belongs to the transforming growth factor-β superfamily and consists of two subunits (α and β) linked by disulphide bonds. It is produced by granulosa cells in the female and Sertoli cells in the male and inhibits pituitary secretion of FSH. A dimer of the β-subunit (activin) stimulates FSH production. Circulating levels of inhibin show peaks at mid-cycle and mid-luteal phase. Inhibin level decrease with age. In pregnancy there is a peak in the first trimester, probably from the corpus luteum, and a second peak towards term.

Control of follicle growth

Initiation of follicular activity does not depend on gonadotrophins and occurs during fetal life and childhood and quiescent periods of adult life such as pregnancy and lactation. Follicles begin development in the same sequence as their arrival as germ cells in the embryonic ovary – the 'first in first out' theory. Follicles containing cells with the greatest number of chiasmata are the first to undergo further development. The regular initiation of growth from the oocyte pool ensures that large numbers of growing follicles are available for further development whenever the appropriate endocrine milieu is present. The time from initiation of growth until ovulation is 85 days.

When follicles reach the 60-cell stage (primary or early secondary follicles of 0.1–0.2 mm), further growth becomes hormone dependent. At the beginning of each menstrual cycle a few primary follicles can respond to gonadotrophins and undergo growth. Ten days before ovulation two or three follicles remain, and by 5 days before only one 'dominant' follicle is usually found.

The action of gonadotrophins on the follicle depends on cell membrane receptors (mol. wt. 20 000–30 000). These receptors have a rapid turnover (half-life 30 min). Only 2% of receptors need to be occupied to initiate a response. FSH receptors are found only in granulosa cells; LH receptors are found on granulosa and theca cells. Oestrogen leads to an increase in FSH receptors, and FSH to an increase in LH receptors. LH depletes gonadotrophin receptors, leading to a refractory period after the LH peak. While both FSH and LH induce follicular growth and steroidogenesis, FSH is more active in the former and LH in the latter respect.

Mechanism of ovulation

The dominant follicle forms a protrusion, the stigma, on the surface of the ovary. The cell layers rupture and the ovum, surrounded by the 'corona radiata' of granulosa cells, is released. The process takes place over about 2 min: it is *not* an instantaneous rupture resulting from a rise in follicular pressure.

Prostaglandin synthesis by granulosa cells increases prior to ovulation and may play a part in the release of collagenase, lysosomal enzymes and plasminogen activator, which may be important in the erosion of the superficial layers of the ovary. (Indomethacin, a prostaglandin inhibitor, blocks ovulation and leads to retention of the oocyte.)

The oocyte and corona are sloughed into follicular fluid shortly before ovulation. This fluid becomes more viscous as ovulation approaches, an important factor in the pick-up of the ovum by fimbriae.

Ovulation is a direct result of the LH surge and occurs some 12 h after the peak of LH values. hCG administered during the late follicular period is followed by ovulation after a remarkably constant 32 h.

The LH surge is thought to be responsible for:

1. Prostaglandin production
2. A decrease in the affinity of gonadotrophin receptors, resulting in desensitisation to LH, and a transient decrease in oestrogens, which may promote subsequent luteinisation
3. Early progesterone secretion
4. Resumption of meiosis by the oocyte

Ovulation appears to alternate between the two ovaries and occurs, on average, 45 days after delivery in non-lactating women; the minimum is 25 days. In lactating women ovulation is unlikely up to 70 days.

Menopausal ovary

Apart from certain strains of rodent, the menopause is confined to the human species and does not occur in other primates. Follicle numbers decline at a steady rate up to age 37, after which there is accelerated loss until the menopause. Several hundred primordial follicles remain in the ovary, but these are insensitive to the action of gonadotrophins and subsequent development is arrested at an early stage.

Oestradiol production is low after the menopause. However, the ovarian stroma continues to secrete androstenedione, and circulating oestrone levels are maintained by peripheral conversion of androstenedione.

Testis

Embryology of the testis

The testis develops in the gonadal ridge after 7 weeks gestation. It descends to the internal inguinal ring during the first trimester (probably under the influence of müllerian inhibiting factor) and through the inguinal canal in the third trimester (probably under the influence of androgens). Differentiation of the testis is directed by a testis-determining factor (TDF) coded on the SRY gene of the Y chromosome. Leydig (interstitial) cells develop rapidly between 12 and 16 weeks and then become less active until birth. The seminiferous tubules consist of Sertoli cells and primitive spermatogonia and remain as solid cords until a lumen forms at 4 or 5 years of age. Sperm are formed continuously from puberty onwards.

Spermatogenesis

The seminiferous tubules have three layers of cells: the spermatogonia, spermatocytes and spermatids. The total thickness is usually six cells. The Sertoli cells lie among the spermatogonia in the basal layer and have processes that extend to the lumen (Fig. 4.7); the spermatids occupy recesses in the apex of these processes. Primitive spermatogonia form type A spermatogonia, which divide mitotically until the primary spermatocyte is formed. This goes through a resting phase and then all the phases of the first meiotic division to form the secondary spermatocytes. The second meiotic division results in formation of spermatids, which are then transformed into mature spermatozoa by the process of spermiogenesis; cytoplasm is lost, nuclear chromatin condenses, the nucleus becomes flattened and the midpiece and flagellum form. The midpiece acquires a cuff of mitochondria, which provide

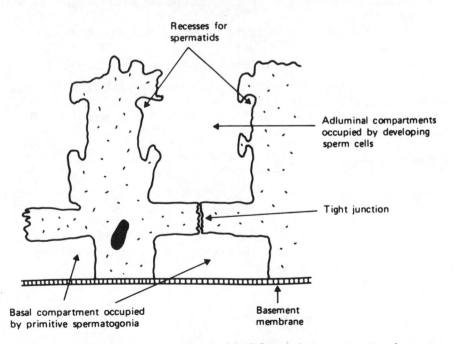

Fig. 4.7. Relationship between Sertoli cells (*shaded*) and the compartments where sperm formation takes place. Sertoli cells divide the seminiferous epithelium into two compartments. The basal compartment contains primitive spermatogonia. Further development takes place in the adluminal compartments, which contain about five layers of germ cells.

the energy for movement. The tail consists of two central singlet microtubules surrounded by nine microtubule doublets and nine outer dense fibres. Side arms of the protein dynein extend from each microtubule; contact between these and adjacent microtubules generates a sliding force and thus movement. The whole process from spermatogonia to mature sperm takes 9–10 weeks. Cytokinesis (division of cytoplasm) does not occur during mitosis or meiosis so that all the progeny of a spermatogonium form a syncytium until release of sperm into the tubule. As a result of this, sperm cells at a given stage of maturation form synchronised groups.

Sertoli cell function

The relationship of Sertoli cells to developing sperm cells is shown in Fig. 4.7. The Sertoli cells (and sperm production) are under the control of FSH. Functions of the Sertoli cells include:

1. Production of an androgen-binding protein (ABP), which is secreted into the seminal plasma. ABP transports testosterone into the seminiferous tubules, where it is partly reduced to dihydrotestosterone and oestrogen. When the ABP–androgen complex reaches the epididymis the ABP is digested enzymatically to yield a high concentration of free androgens.

2. Production of intracellular and androgen-binding receptor.

3. Conversion of testosterone to oestradiol (50% of E_2 in males comes from the testis).

4. Transport of fully formed sperm cells into the lumen (involving a system of microtubules and microfilaments).

5. Production of inhibin, which has a negative feedback on FSH.

Fetal Sertoli cells secrete Müllerian inhibiting factor (MIF), which causes involution of the Müllerian ducts in the male fetus. MIF is a glycoprotein related to inhibin. Small amounts are also found in adult granulosa cells.

Sperm transport

Sperm are carried passively along the seminiferous tubules by contraction of surrounding muscle cells. Full maturity is reached in the epididymis, but the spermatozoa do not become motile until they have left this site because of a local inhibitory factor. Sperm are carried along the vas deferens and most of them are stored in this duct rather than the seminal vesicles, which have a predominantly secretory function.

Sperm can appear in the pouch of Douglas within 30 min of deposition in the vagina.

Ejaculate

The average ejaculate consists of 2–5 ml of seminal fluid with a sperm density of 60 million/ml.

Composition of seminal plasma

A number of materials are secreted directly into the seminal plasma and are therefore at relatively high concentrations in this site. These include fructose and citric acid (seminal vesicles); inositol, carnitine and glycerophosphocholine (epididymis); acid phosphatases (prostate); and a number of 'placental' proteins (source unknown).

Leydig cell function

In the male, 95% of testosterone synthesis occurs in Leydig cells, which occur in clusters at the angles between seminiferous tubules. The very high local concentration of testosterone stimulates spermatogenesis, the effect being mediated via the Sertoli cells. Most of the testosterone is produced by the Δ4-pathway via progesterone (Fig. 4.6a). Circulating levels show a circadian rhythm, with maximal levels in the morning. Production of testosterone is under the control of LH, with a negative feedback at the hypothalamus and pituitary. FSH elevation precedes that of LH at puberty, and the former increases the sensitivity of Leydig cells to the action of LH. Testosterone levels fall slowly after the age of 50.

Congenital abnormalities of androgen function

Testicular feminisation.   This is a familial condition in which the intracellular androgen receptor protein is absent or defective. The patient has a male karyotype, normal female external genitalia and no internal genitalia apart from intra-abdominal testes. Lesser degrees of the condition are associated with a normal male phenotype but an absence of sperm production (Reifenstein's syndrome).

α-Reductase deficiency.   In this familial condition, the patient has a male karyotype, female external genitalia and male internal genitalia (ejaculatory ducts terminate in a blind-ending vagina). There are two 5α-reductase genes. One of these is the major isozyme in genital tissue and is defective in some cases of male pseudohermaphroditism.

Thyroid gland

The thyroid gland secretes two iodine-containing hormones, thyroxine (T_4) and tri-iodothyronine (T_3), and the peptide calcitonin.

Anatomy

Four weeks after conception the thyroid develops as a thickening in the floor of the pharynx. It passes down the front of the neck, at first being connected to the pharynx by the thyroglossal duct, and divides into two lobes separated by an isthmus.

The gland contains 1 million follicles, each consisting of a single layer of cells surrounding a colloidal fluid. Numerous microvilli line the apical surface of the cells and protrude into the colloid. The follicular cells function in three ways:

1. *Exocrine*: secreting products into the follicular lumen
2. *Absorptive*: pinocytosing these secretions back into the cell
3. *Endocrine*: secreting hormones directly into the blood

Chemistry and metabolism

T_3 and T_4 are formed by iodination of the amino acid tyrosine. Monoiodotyrosine (MIT) and diiodotyrosine (DIT) are formed by the addition of one or two iodine atoms to the tyrosine molecule. Two molecules of DIT combine to form T_4, and T_3 is formed from one molecule of MIT and one of DIT. In each case an alanine molecule is released.

The events leading to thyroid hormone secretion are:

1. Iodine 'trapping' (Fig. 4.8). Iodine is absorbed and circulates in the blood as inorganic iodide – about 150μg (1000 nmol) per day is required. Iodide is cleared by the thyroid; the thyroid:serum ratio is about 25:1, rising to 250:1 in iodine deficiency. The iodine 'pumps' are blocked by perchlorate and thiocyanate, which compete with iodide for the carrier mechanism.

2. Oxidation of iodide in the microvilli by a membrane-bound peroxidase releasing free iodine at the cell–colloid interface. This is blocked by propylthiouracil and carbimazole.

3. Synthesis of thyroglobulin (a glycoprotein, mol. wt. 660 000) on ribosomes and storage in vesicles which are extruded by exocytosis (reverse pinocytosis) (Fig. 4.9).

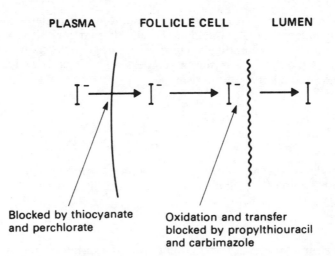

Fig. 4.8. Iodide is cleared from the plasma and transferred to the luminal surface of the thyroid cell. Here it is oxidised to iodine and transferred to the lumen. Iodide is also released during intracellular de-iodination of excess T_3 and T_4.

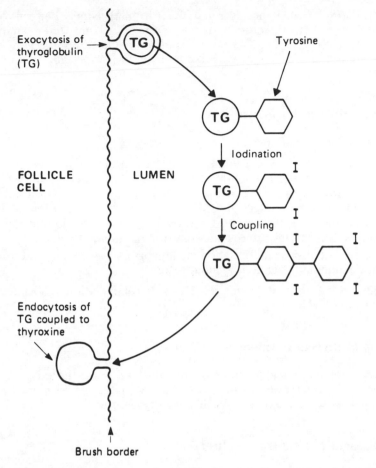

Fig. 4.9. Iodination of tyrosine takes place on the thyroglobulin molecule in the lumen to form monoiodotyrosine and diiodotyrosine. Diiodotyrosine 'couples' with either monoiodotyrosine (to form T_3) or another molecule of diiodotyrosine (to form T_4).

4. Attachment of tyrosine molecules by peptide linkages to the thyroglobulin molecules in the lumen. Iodine attaches to the tyrosyl groups.

5. Coupling of iodotyrosines to form T_3 and T_4. These remain attached to thyroglobulin, which constitutes a storage depot.

6. Ingestion of colloid by pinocytosis followed by proteolysis in lysosomes to release T_4 and T_3 (secreted in a ratio of 20–30 : 1, the proportion of T_3 being increased in iodine deficiency). Some 99.5% of circulating thyroid hormones are protein bound, leaving a small biologically active fraction: T_4 is bound 10 times more avidly than T_3. Seventy-five per cent of both hormones are bound to thyroxine-binding globulin (TBG) (an α_2-globulin, mol. wt. 60 000); 15% of T_4 (but not T_3) is bound to thyroxine-binding pre-albumin; and 10% of T_4 and 25% of T_3 is bound to albumin.

Free T_4 and T_3 are de-iodinated in cells throughout the body. In this process T_4 is converted to T_3 and free iodide is excreted in the urine or recirculated (some 20% of T_3 and T_4 are excreted intact in bile). Ninety per cent of T_3 is derived by peripheral de-iodination of T_4. Some T_4 is converted to an inactive isomer of T_3, 'reverse T_3'. The reverse T_3 level is increased in severe illness, in starvation and after major surgery; reverse T_3 is especially prominent in the fetus.

Action of thyroid hormones

The actions of thyroid hormones include:

1. Increase of oxygen consumption and heat production (increased basal metabolic rate, BMR). These effects have a long latent period: after thyroid-ectomy the BMR halves over 30 days; administration of T_4 has no effect for 24 h and the maximum effect on BMR is only reached after 10 days. Tissues that do not increase oxygen consumption in response to thyroid hormones are brain, spleen, testes, uterus and anterior pituitary.

2. Increase of glucose mobilisation via glycogenolysis; increase of free fatty acid production and decrease in cholesterol.

Deficiency of thyroid hormones leads to anovulation associated with increased LH levels.

Control of thyroid hormone secretion

Pituitary TSH promotes synthesis of thyroid hormones; there is a negative feedback of T_4 exerted at the pituitary level. TSH-releasing hormone from the hypothalamus stimulates the TSH-thyroid response to stimuli such as cold.

Development of fetal thyroid function

Very little maternal T_3 and T_4 cross the placenta. However, iodine is actively transferred by the placenta, and fetal thyroid function begins at 10 weeks. Relatively more reverse T_3 is manufactured in peripheral tissues, especially in early pregnancy. TSH reaches a peak between 20 and 30 weeks of fetal life and then decreases, but is still above adult levels at birth. T_4 secretion increases rapidly between 20 and 30 weeks and continues to rise more slowly to term, although levels are always less than maternal. In amniotic fluid T_4 is higher because of the lower concentration of TBG. After birth TSH increases again, returning to normal adult levels by 3 days. Lack of thyroid hormones produces deficiency in skeletal and cerebral maturation characteristic of cretinism, and pulmonary surfactant production is delayed. Postnatally, thyroid deficiency severely impairs skeletal growth, leading to dwarfism. Most of the cerebral consequences of cretinism can be forestalled by replacement therapy.

Maternal thyroid in pregnancy

Iodine loss in urine due to the increased glomerular filtration rate leads to a reduction in serum iodide and an increase in the size and vascularity of the gland. TBG levels increase under the influence of oestrogen in the first trimester and remain at high levels until term. Total T_4 and T_3 are increased, and the total daily production of these hormones is increased. Free T_4 and T_3 are unchanged or marginally decreased, though there is a transient increase in free T_4 in the first trimester owing to the thyrotrophic effect of hCG. If dietary iodine is adequate, TSH remains normal or only slightly increased. The TSH response to TSH-releasing hormone is slightly increased (an oestrogen effect). Serum thyroglobulin levels increase.

Adrenal cortex

The adrenal cortex comprises three morphologically and functionally distinct regions. The outermost region (zona glomerulosa) secretes aldosterone. The zona reticularis encircles the medulla and synthesises oestrogens and androgens. The zona fasciculata is intermediate and produces cortisol. In the fetus the gland consists mainly of the fetal zone, which is surrounded by the definitive layers and begins to atrophy shortly before birth.

The adrenal cortex develops from cells of the coelomic mesoderm near the anterior pole of the mesonephros. The adrenal medulla arises from ectodermal cells from the neural crests.

The synthetic pathways for steroid production are outlined in Fig. 4.6. Cortisol and corticosterone bind to corticosteroid-binding globulin (CBG) and with less affinity to albumin. Around 10% is in the biologically active free form. Protein binding of aldosterone is very weak.

Control of glucocorticoid secretion

The secretion of cortisol is controlled exclusively by ACTH. ACTH also promotes glucose uptake and increases blood-flow in the adrenal. Glucocorticoids suppress ACTH secretion, acting at both the hypothalamic *and* the pituitary level. The feedback has two components: fast feedback, which is mediated by the rate of change of cortisol levels and prevents ACTH *release*, and slow feedback, which is dependent on the absolute levels and influences ACTH *synthesis*.

The hypothalamus controls ACTH secretion predominantly by means of corticotrophin-releasing hormone (CRH), although vasopressin also increases ACTH release. CRH itself is controlled by circadian factors. Thus, cortisol secretion is maximal at around 6 a.m. Stress also increases cortisol secretion via release of CRH. The placenta secretes CRH and there is a dramatic increase in maternal CRH in the last 8 weeks of pregnancy.

Control of mineralocorticoid secretion

The most important factor controlling aldosterone secretion is angiotensin. Renin from the juxtaglomerular cells in the kidney cleaves angiotensinogen (an α_2-globulin from the liver) to yield the decapeptide angiotensin I. A pulmonary converting enzyme cleaves two further amino acids to yield angiotensin II.

The juxtaglomerular cells are specialised endothelial cells in the afferent arteriole of the glomerulus. They are closely related to the macula densa, which is a region of tubule cells at the point where the distal convoluted tubule bends back near its own glomerulus.

Renin is derived from an inactive precursor form, prorenin. Renin release is stimulated by: (a) decreased renal perfusion (e.g. hypotension or renal artery stenosis), (b) decreased extracellular fluid volume (e.g. dehydration), (c) sodium depletion (e.g. congenital adrenal hyperplasia or diuretic treatment), and (d) β-adrenergic drugs (which constrict the afferent arteriole). Prorenin is also secreted by ovarian follicles. Circulating prorenin increases at mid-cycle and in response to stimulation with LH or hCG.

ACTH has a 'permissive' effect on the zona glomerulosa by ensuring a supply of precursors for aldosterone. Large amounts of ACTH released in severe stress have a direct stimulatory effect on aldosterone secretion.

Control of sex steroid secretion

Sex steroid secretion is promoted by ACTH, but other, unknown, factors must bring about the increase in androgen production (adrenarche) that precedes puberty.

Actions of glucocorticoids

The effects of glucocorticoids on various tissues are summarised in Table 4.6. Normal levels of cortisol are also necessary for optimal growth. Excessive cortisol diminishes growth by its general catabolic effect, whereas inadequate cortisol does so by decreased appetite and intestinal absorption.

Maternal adrenal cortex during pregnancy

The total amount of cortisol in the blood increases, as does that of the binding globulin. There is an increase in the free fraction of cortisol and in the urinary excretion of cortisol. ACTH level rises throughout pregnancy, although it may initially decrease in the first trimester. The pigmentary changes that occur in pregnancy are probably the result of this increase in ACTH (α-MSH is not thought to exist in free form in human blood). The circadian rhythms of ACTH (and thus cortisol) persist during pregnancy, and a considerable increase occurs with the stress of labour. Renin substrate, renin and aldosterone levels all increase during pregnancy.

Congenital adrenal hyperplasia

This is a group of autosomal recessive syndromes resulting from defects in the enzyme steps of adrenal steroidogenesis (Fig. 4.6b). The commonest defect is of 21-hydroxylase, in which there is failure of conversion of progesterone and 17α-hydroxyprogesterone to 11-deoxycorticosterone (DOC) and 22-deoxycortisol. There is therefore a deficiency of cortisol and aldosterone.

Table 4.6. Summary of the peripheral actions of glucocorticoids

Tissue	Action
Liver	Increases gluconeogenesis from amino acids
Skeletal muscle	Normal amounts required for efficient contractility. Excessive amounts lead to protein catabolism, to diminished glucose uptake due to presence of excessive free fatty acids, and to muscle atrophy
Adipose tissue	An anti-insulin effect diminishes glucose uptake. Increased release of free fatty acids
Peripheral blood vessels	Potentiates vasoconstrictor effects of catecholamines
Nervous system	Depression in deficiency, euphoria in excess
Lymphoid tissue	Normal amounts cause thymic regression in infancy and prevent excessive growth of lymphoid tissues. Excessive amounts cause dissolution of lymphoid tissue, reduction in plasma and mast cell proliferation, lymphopenia and impaired phagocytosis and lysosome activity
Ground substance	Cortisol inhibits mucopolysaccharide synthesis and increases fluid accumulation. Inhibits development of fibroblasts
Pituitary/hypothalamus	Inhibits ACTH secretion
Kidney	Increases sodium reabsorption (1/500th as effective as aldosterone)
Placenta	Increases oestrogen and decreases progesterone production. This leads to parturition in some species but not in humans
Fetal lung	Cortisol is responsible for the surge in surfactant production in the middle of the third trimester. It also causes a more stable form of surfactant to be produced – diphosphoglycerocholine

In turn, this stimulates ACTH and MSH and thus produces an increase in androgens (Fig. 4.6b). The newborn female is masculinised. In the severest cases there is salt loss and adrenal insufficiency. The diagnostic feature is elevation of plasma 17α-hydroxyprogesterone, its urinary metabolite, pregnanetriol, and plasma renin.

1. *11-Hydroxylase deficiency*: similar to 21-hydroxylase deficiency, but large amounts of mineralocorticoid DOC are formed (see Fig. 4.6b); salt loss does not occur and hypertension is sometimes a feature.

2. *17α-Hydroxylase deficiency*: prevents formation of cortisol and all sex steroids but not mineralocorticoids (Fig. 4.6b).

3. *3β-Hydroxysteroid dehydrogenase deficiency*: blocks the corticosteroid, mineralocorticoid and main sex steroid pathways (Fig. 4.6b). Elevated dehydroepiandrosterone (Δ5-pathway) may cause partial virilisation.

The gene for 21-hydroxylation is located among the HLA genes on chromosome 6 and is known as CYP21B. In one-quarter of cases of adrenal hyperplasia both CYP21B genes are deleted. In the remaining three-quarters there is substitution of an abnormal amino acid in the amino acid sequence.

Adrenal medulla

The adrenal medulla arises from neural crest cells and makes up 10% of the gland. The synthetic pathway of its products, the catecholamines, is shown in Fig. 4.10. These products are stored and released as granules. The principal urinary excretory product of the catecholamines is vanillylmandelic acid (VMA).

Catecholamines are also widely distributed in other tissues (associated with their sympathetic innervation), but are absent from the bone marrow and placenta. However, conversion of noradrenaline to adrenaline occurs almost exclusively in the adrenal medulla; thus adrenalectomy leads to a fall in circulating adrenaline but no change in noradrenaline. In the fetus and neonate there are substantial amounts of catecholamines in the organ of Zuckerkandl and the extramedullary chromaffin tissue.

A variety of stressful stimuli cause an increase in circulating catecholamines, including exercise, insulin hypoglycaemia, hypoxia, haemorrhage and hypotension. There is no change in circulating noradrenaline levels in the mother during pregnancy.

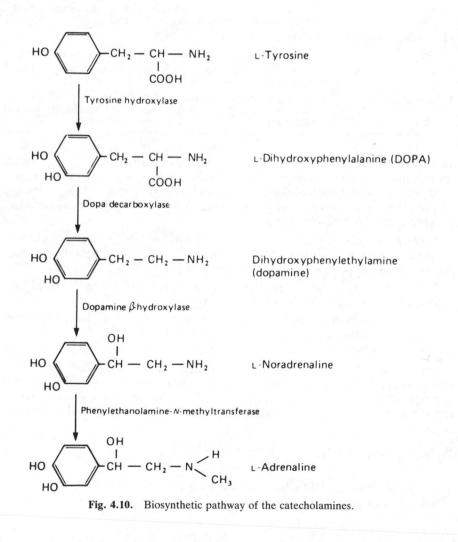

Fig. 4.10. Biosynthetic pathway of the catecholamines.

Adrenaline stimulates both α- and β-receptors in tissues, whereas noradrenaline acts only on the α-receptors. Thus, noradrenaline constricts while adrenaline dilates the skeletal muscle arterioles. Both cause constriction of skin and gut arterioles. Via β-receptors, adrenaline relaxes the smooth muscle of the gastrointestinal tract, bronchioles, bladder and uterus. In addition, it increases glycogen breakdown in the liver and muscle and increases lipolysis in fat.

The main catecholamine in fetal plasma and amniotic fluid is L-dopa. Dopamine and noradrenaline levels in amniotic fluid increase dramatically in late pregnancy.

Hormones involved in calcium homeostasis

These include parathormone, secreted by the parathyroid glands (84 amino acids, mol. wt. 9500); calcitonin, secreted by C cells, a group of parafollicular cells scattered throughout the thyroid (32 amino acids, mol. wt. 3200); and vitamin D. Vitamin D is a prohormone, which may be derived from the diet or from the effect of sunlight on cholesterol derivatives in the skin. A sequence of hydroxylations, beginning in the liver and ending in the kidney, lead to the production of the active hormone 1,25-dihydrocholecalciferol.

Parathormone (PTH) increases circulating calcium by a number of mechanisms, including enhanced renal calcium reabsorption, increased intestinal calcium absorption and mobilisation of calcium from bone. The effect on the gut is indirect, being mediated by PTH-induced synthesis of 1,25-dihydrocholecalciferol in the kidney. Secretion of PTH is controlled mainly by plasma ionised calcium; magnesium has a similar but less important effect.

Calcitonin decreases circulating calcium by inhibiting bone resorption; like PTH, it is controlled by the level of ionised calcium and phosphorus. Levels of calcitonin are lower in women than in men, and in both sexes the levels fall with age. Both oestrogens and testosterone stimulate calcitonin secretion.

Vitamin D hormones increase circulating calcium and phosphorus and enhance bone mineralisation; renal synthesis is controlled by calcium, phosphorus and PTH.

The fetal parathyroids are active from the 12th week of gestation. PTH levels are lower in the fetus than in the mother, and secretion rises sharply at days 2–7 of neonatal life. Calcitonin levels are higher in the fetus than in the mother and show a further rise in the first 48 h of neonatal life. The role and origin of vitamin D in the fetus are uncertain, although congenital rickets may occur in the infants of vitamin D-deficient mothers.

During pregnancy maternal levels of vitamin D are normal, while those of PTH, calcitonin and 1,25-dihydrocholecalciferol are elevated. The latter is due, in part, to placental production. After the menopause there is a fall in the levels of all calcium-controlling hormones.

Puberty

The first signs of puberty are an acceleration of growth and appearance of the breast bud (telarche). This is followed by the appearance of pubic hair and then, after a further 2 years, axillary hair starts to grow. Menarche is a late event, occurring after the peak of the growth spurt has been passed.

The adolescent growth spurt of the typical girl occurs 2 years earlier than that of boys, but is less marked. The peak growth rate for British girls (6–11 cm in a year) is reached at the age of 12. The mean age of menarche is 13. Early cycles are often anovulatory and therefore irregular and sometimes heavy.

Puberty in girls is associated with nocturnal pulses of LH (REM sleep). The amplitude increases as puberty progresses but daytime pulses are not seen until after menarche. The nocturnal pulse is followed by an increase in circulating oestrogens. These endocrine changes are primarily dependent on release of GnRH; puberty is associated with an increase in GnRH pulse frequency. The latter may in turn be controlled by pineal indoles and body weight. The increased gonadal activity is preceded by increased androgen production, first dehydroepiandrosterone at age 6–8 years and then androstenedione at 8–10 years; these hormones are responsible for pubic and axillary hair growth. Multicystic ovaries are apparent by 8 years. Adrenarche is not, however, an essential part of puberty. Random short-lived spikes of progesterone secretion occur before menarche and during early anovulatory cycles.

Menopause

The menopause is the last menstrual period. The average age at which this occurs is 50–51 in the UK. The period leading up to the menopause is the climacteric and it is characterised by increasing frequency of anovulatory cycles.

The ovarian changes have been described. All other structural changes in the reproductive tract are entirely secondary to declining oestrogen (especially E_2) secretion. Atrophy occurs in the vulva and vagina with loss of superficial glycogen-containing cells. The endometrium is thin and the body of the uterus becomes smaller in comparison to the cervix. Systemic sequelae of oestrogen deficiency include accelerated osteoporosis and perhaps an increased risk of coronary artery disease and psychiatric disorders.

Hormonal patterns preceding the menopause

Changes in gonadotrophins are very variable over the years preceding the menopause. Both tend to rise and the increase in FSH is usually, but not invariably, greater than that in LH. There is considerable intra- and inter-cycle variation in gonadotrophin levels. Levels are usually higher in the follicular phase of the cycle and vary from typical menopausal levels in some cycles to 'normal' reproductive levels in others. The luteal phase is often shorter and progesterone levels decline with age.

Table 4.7. A classification of materials and processes which may be involved in the initiation of parturition

Classification	Examples
Type 1	Fetal oxytocin, ACTH and related peptides
Type 2	Oestrogen, progesterone, cortisol, maternal oxytocin, oxytocin receptors, relaxin
Type 3	Prostaglandins, autonomic mediators, calcium, gap junctions, cyclic nucleotides

Type 1 includes factors which might constitute a primary stimulus to labour. Type 2 factors are fairly specific to parturition but are dependent on a primary stimulus. Type 3 factors are non-specific and are involved in the activation of smooth muscle at any site

Hormonal patterns after the menopause

Gonadotrophin secretion is persistently raised and maximal levels are reached after 2–3 years. FSH values reach 13 times early proliferative phase levels and LH values are 5 times greater. These high levels gradually decline over the following years. Gonadotrophin pulses occur with the same frequency as in the follicular phase, but the amplitude is much greater. Vasomotor symptoms are associated with, but not caused by, these pulses. The net LH and FSH response to GnRH is also increased. Prolactin levels fall after the menopause.

Oestradiol, androstenedione and DHEA levels are considerably lower after the menopause, but E_1 levels are about the same as those found in the early follicular phase of the cycle. The ovary makes a relatively small contribution to postmenopausal oestrogen secretion. It does, however, secrete increased amounts of testosterone owing to stromal stimulation by high levels of gonadotrophins. Total testosterone levels are nevertheless slightly lower because of decreased peripheral conversion of androstenedione, but free testosterone level increases owing to lower SHBG levels. Oestrone levels are maintained by peripheral conversion of androstenedione in fat and skin; most of this androstenedione is of adrenal origin.

Initiation of labour

The basic trigger for human labour is still unknown, but is believed to reside with the fetus rather than the mother. Numerous factors may be involved (Table 4.7).

There is no sudden change in type 2 and 3 factors prior to the onset of labour, but type 1 factors may constitute the primary event. Pregnancy is sometimes prolonged in the absence of the fetal pituitary (anencephaly) and a specific role has been suggested for fetal oxytocin and for ACTH and ACTH-related peptides. This effect is not mediated by cortisol in the human, and the rise in cortisol levels during labour is due to stress. Labour appears to be a self-perpetuating process once initiated, and type 2 and 3 factors are particularly important in this respect. For example, during labour there is an increase in 'spurt' release of maternal oxytocin, probably stimulated by a neural reflex arising from distension of the lower genital tract (Ferguson's reflex). Type 3 factors, including prostaglandins, are activated from the decidua and myometrium during the course of labour. The rate-limiting step is release of arachidonic acid by phospholipase, and this enzyme is activated in the early stages of labour.

An important factor in the onset of labour is softening of the cervix due to decreased affinity of glycosaminoglycans for collagen and increasing hydration of the ground substance.

Pineal gland

This is a neuroendocrine transducer situated at the posterior end of the third ventricle. It is innervated by a sympathetic pathway originating in the retina and reaching the gland via the lateral horn of the spinal cord, cervical ganglia and carotid plexus. During darkness the gland secretes a range of indole hormones derived from serotonin. The best known of these is melatonin. Melatonin inhibits gonadotrophin secretion in seasonal breeders but not in humans.

Atrial natriuretic peptide (ANP)

ANP is a 28-amino-acid peptide synthesised principally by the cardiac atria. It increases excretion of sodium and water and is involved in the control of blood volume. It also relaxes vascular smooth muscle and decreases blood-pressure.

Chapter 5

Pathology

Inflammation

Acute inflammation

Acute inflammation is the local response of living tissue to injury; the latter
may include trauma, chemicals, radiation, vascular necrosis, heat and cold,
organisms and antigen–antibody reactions. It includes a vascular response,
formation of an exudate, and other changes.

The earliest vascular response is constriction of small vessels, rapidly
followed by dilatation and a brief increase in the velocity of blood-flow. The
endothelial lining becomes swollen and sticky, with adherence of leucocytes
(margination of polymorphs) and platelets; red cells aggregate as rouleaux
and the combination of events leads to slowing of blood-flow (sludging).

The exudate includes fluid and cells. Increased permeability of the capillary
endothelium, together with increased capillary pressure and fluidity of tissue
ground substance, leads to leakage of fluid with the same composition as
plasma (normally only water and electrolytes pass freely). The permeability
change may be associated with widening of the gaps between endothelial cells.
The exudate contains immunoglobulins and other antibacterial factors as well
as fibrinogen, which may form a fibrin clot.

White cells also emigrate (diapedesis) through the endothelial gaps. The
first cells involved are neutrophil polymorphs. Later the blood monocytes
predominate and become phagocytic (macrophages). Lymphocytes are not
involved in the acute phase. The phagocytosis of virulent organisms, whether
by polymorphs or monocytes, depends on serum factors known as opsonins
and also on activation of complement. The cell energy requirements for
phagocytosis are met by anaerobic glycolysis, and in polymorphs there are
dramatic increases in the hexose monophosphate shunt and in NADPH. In
the process of phagocytosis, particles are ingested in a vacuole, which then
fuses with lysosomes to form a digestion vacuole.

Another early feature of inflammation is degranulation of mast cells in
adjacent tissues, with release of histamine and heparin.

Table 5.1. Chemical factors that may be involved in acute inflammation. The relative contribution of individual factors is poorly understood

Factor	Source	Probable action
Histamine	Mast cells	Early vascular response
5-Hydroxytryptamine	–	Early vascular response
Kinins[a]	–	Vasodilatation, pain
Complement[b]	Plasma	–
Prostaglandins	?Platelets	Later phases of reaction
Nucleosides	–	–
Bacterial toxins		
Leukotrienes (slow reactive substance A)	Leucocytes	Smooth muscle contribution; chemotaxis
Cytokines (especially interleukins)		
Growth factors		

[a] Kinins are polypeptides that cause contraction of smooth muscle (e.g. bradykinin, kallidin) and are involved in local and general pain mechanisms (tachykinins, e.g. substance P). They are formed as a result of the action of various enzymes on precursor molecules; the enzymes include kallikrein, globulin permeability factor and plasmin.

[b] Complement components may act as chemotactic agents, attracting white cells to particles such as bacteria.

Subsequent events depend on the cause and extent of the inflammation. In the phase of *demolition,* macrophages engulf fibrin, red cells, pus cells, bacteria, etc. The complete return to normal is referred to as *resolution.* If there is substantial tissue necrosis (as with staphylococcal lesions or chemical agents such as turpentine), the process of autolysis leads to the formation of pus (dead cells and cell debris, etc.) contained within a cavity to form an abscess.

Chemical factors are involved in acute inflammation (Table 5.1). In addition, the liver produces increased amounts of C-reactive protein in response to inflammation elsewhere in the body.

Chronic inflammation

Chronic inflammation is defined as a prolonged process in which destruction and inflammation are taking place at the same time as healing. The causes are damaging agents that persist beyond the stage of the acute response (e.g. foreign bodies, organisms (tuberculosis and actinomycosis) and collagen diseases) or delayed healing.

The histology varies with the cause and may include elements of acute inflammation, demolition and healing. In chronic suppurative inflammation (abscess) polymorphs abound. In other circumstances there is an abundance of macrophages or epithelioid cells: this is typical of tuberculosis (TB) and other conditions (e.g. sarcoidosis, lupus vulgaris and leprosy) and may include caseation (a central solid mass of inert debris). When macrophages encounter insoluble material they frequently coalesce to form giant cells (e.g. Langhans' giant cells in TB). Chronic inflammation may lead to the formation of a solid tumour-like mass or *granuloma,* in which macrophages predominate. These are typical of infections such as TB, syphilis (the gumma), yaws, leprosy and actinomycosis; of reactions to foreign bodies (talc granuloma); and of certain collagen diseases (Wegener's granulomatosis).

Other features of chronic inflammation may include evidence of a healing process (migration of capillaries and fibroblasts, and formation of collagen); occlusion of small arteries by intimal proliferation (endarteritis obliterans); accumulation of lymphocytes and plasma cells in perivascular areas (e.g. syphilitic aortitis); and excessive growth of regenerating normal tissues (polypoid growths in ulcerative colitis).

General effects of chronic inflammation include a proliferative response in the reticuloendothelial system, especially local and regional lymph nodes; immune responses, which may be sufficient to elevate total IgG levels in blood (kala-azar) and are sometimes associated with cellular delayed hypersensitivity (Mantoux, Frei and lepromin tests); and changes in blood cells (anaemia, raised erythrocyte sedimentation rate and raised white cell count, especially lymphocytes and monocytes).

Examples

Osteomyelitis occurs at the metaphysis of long bones and is the result of blood-borne spread of *Staphylococcus pyogenes*. The acute phase leads to extensive necrosis and pus formation, and thereby a chronic infection.

Chronic pyelonephritis is caused by infection by Gram-negative intestinal bacilli (e.g. *E. coli*), leading to the formation of multiple small abscesses in the renal cortex. The origin and chronic nature are usually based on urinary obstruction.

Ulcerative colitis may be due to infections such as *Shigella* or *Entamoeba histolytica*, but the commonest form is idiopathic. Acute inflammation leads to blockage of the opening of the crypts of Lieberkuhn, with formation of small abscesses; tissue necrosis causes ulceration and even perforation. The mucosa is oedematous and infiltrated with lymphocytes; hypertrophy of the muscle coat occurs but fibrosis is a minor feature.

Tuberculosis. The most characteristic lesion is the tubercle follicle with an area of caseation (necrotic debris) surrounded by macrophages (epithelioid cells) in turn surrounded by a zone of lymphocytes and fibroblasts.

Amyloid disease

Amyloid is an unusual complication of chronic infection, collagen disease and multiple myeloma (10%). There is an extracellular deposit around small blood vessels of β-pleated sheets of protein fibrils, principally affecting the liver, spleen and kidneys. The deposit stains strongly with Congo red and shows an apple-green birefringence in polarised light. The amyloid protein is coded by chromosome 21. In cases of myeloma the deposit contains immunoglobulin light chains; in inflammatory conditions it contains the acute phase reactant protein, serum amyloid A (SAA). Cerebrovascular deposits of amyloid are found in Alzheimer's disease and in older individuals with Down's syndrome.

Wound healing

Immediately after a wound is made the defect fills with blood and a fibrin clot is formed; there is an acute inflammatory reaction in adjacent tissue. The subsequent process of healing for a clean wound of the skin includes a lag phase and a repair phase.

In the *lag phase* there is a progressive accumulation of enzymes in the vicinity of the wound: esterase, adenosine triphosphatase, aminopeptidase and phosphatases. There is a vascular and cellular response similar to inflammation. After transitory vasoconstriction there is vasodilatation of the small vessels, increased permeability of the endothelium and exudation of plasma. Polymorph and mononuclear white cells enter the exudate by diapedesis.

The *repair phase* begins within a few days and includes contraction, fibroplasia and epidermal ingrowth. Contraction is due to shortening of newly formed collagen fibres and the activity of myofibroblasts. Fibroplasia is associated with budding of adjacent capillaries (solid endothelial buds which then become canalised) and migration of fibroblasts and phagocytes into the wound cavity, thus forming vascular *granulation tissue*. The fibroblasts synthesise collagen and mucopolysaccharides, which increasingly strengthen the tissue; eventually the fibrous scar becomes relatively acellular and avascular. Healthy epidermal cells at the wound margins migrate down the sides of the wound and across the granulation and fibrous tissues, a process involving both movement of the cells and division to form new cells in the basal layer of the epidermis near the wound margin. The process is terminated by contact inhibition between epidermal cells when coverage is complete. The limit of epithelial ingrowth is 1 cm from the wound margin.

In the fetus skin wounds heal without scarring.

Tensile strength and elasticity of a healing wound

The tensile strength depends on the amount and arrangement of collagen fibres. Collagen content of a wound is maximal at 80 days, but the strength may not reach a maximum for many months.

The elasticity of the skin depends on elastin fibres in the dermis arranged in parallel with skin creases. Incisions across creases (Langer's lines) tend to gape and heal less well than those parallel to creases.

Local factors in wound healing

1. *Vascularity*: Highly vascular areas (face, scalp) heal faster than less vascular areas (trunk and limbs).

2. *Separation*: A clean skin wound with neatly apposed edges will heal rapidly with minimal granulation (healing by primary intention). A wound with separated edges will take longer (healing by secondary intention), although the basic process is the same.

3. *Necrosis*: Necrosis at wound margins delays repair.

4. *Lymph drainage*: Impairment of lymph drainage causes oedema and delays repair.

5. *Movement*: This delays repair and predisposes to stretching and keloid formation.

6. *Foreign bodies*: Unless inert (stainless steel and certain plastics), these can cause inflammation and delay repair. Catgut sutures are notable irritants, chromic catgut rather less so, plastic and silk much less so (although the latter are non-absorbable and may act as a nidus for bacterial infection).

7. *Infection*: This is the most common and important factor that delays repair.

Systemic factors in wound healing

1. *Protein*: Deficiency delays wound repair, especially of sulphur-containing amino acids such as methionine.

2. *Vitamin C* (ascorbic acid): Deficiency (scurvy or malabsorption) leads to failure of collagen formation (conversion of proline to hydroxyproline).

3. *Corticosteroids*: These can delay healing, but only if high doses are given for prolonged periods.

4. *Zinc*: Experimental zinc deficiency impairs strength of scars.

5. *Temperature*: Wounds heal more slowly at low temperatures.

Wound healing in tissues other than skin

The basic process of initial haemorrhage and inflammation, formation of granulation tissue, and eventual fibroplasia is the same in all sites. However, repair of specialised cells is variable:

1. *Bone*: Proliferation of osteoblasts, formation of collagen and osteomucin, and calcification lead to formation of woven bone. Subsequently, the new tissue is reorganised by the combined action of osteoblasts and osteoclasts to form lamellar bone.

2. *Lining epithelia* (e.g. gut): Similar to skin. Specialised structures (e.g. villi, glands, cilia) are recreated.

3. *Liver*: Remaining cells proliferate to replace damaged tissue.

4. *Kidney*: Tubules can regenerate; glomeruli cannot.

5. *Muscle* (smooth and striated): Muscle cells can regenerate from myoblasts (satellite cells), but this ability is very limited and union is usually through scar tissue.

6. *Nervous tissue*: Adult nerve cells cannot divide or regenerate. If the

axon is divided, neurofibrils may sprout from the proximal cut end and migrate distally along the path of the original Schwann cells at a rate of 1 mm/day.

Metabolic response to injury

There is a sequence of events which may follow any major trauma (e.g. surgery). The immediate response (fight or flight reaction) includes increased output of adrenaline and noradrenaline, peripheral vasoconstriction, a rise of diastolic blood pressure and pulse rate, release of cortisol, quickening of reaction times, and release of glucose. Subsequent events can be divided under the headings of catabolic response, fluid conservation and mobilisation of energy resources.

Catabolic response

The cortisol (pituitary–adrenal) response to trauma may be prolonged. Nitrogen excretion in urine increases from 5–10 g/day to 25 g/day. This is mainly urea derived from cell proteins, but also incudes creatinine from muscle. Potassium excretion in urine greatly increases, and during the first week may total 100–300 mmol; if renal function is normal the potassium is rapidly excreted with little elevation of the blood level. Blood urea levels above 300 mg% or potassium levels above 7 mg% suggest the need for dialysis.

Fluid conservation

Acute blood loss may lead to peripheral vasodilatation, hypotension and fainting. This is rapidly followed by a widespread sympathetic vasoconstriction of arterioles and veins. If compensation is inadequate, the fall in blood volume leads to impaired filling of the right atrium: blood pressure falls despite reflex tachycardia. Reduced hydrostatic pressure in capillaries leads to a shift of fluid from tissues into the bloodstream. The compensatory mechanism takes 24 h to complete and leads to a progressive fall in red cell count. Replacement of plasma proteins takes 2–3 days, and that of red cells 6 weeks (in the absence of transfusion).

There is release of antidiuretic hormone (ADH, vasopressin), which promotes reabsorption of water from distal tubules, and of renin/aldosterone, which promotes sodium reabsorption in the same site. As a result, the volume and sodium content of urine may fall drastically in the first 24 h (although specific gravity remains above 1.015 unless there is renal damage). The reduction in sodium bicarbonate excretion may cause a mild alkalosis which, by shifting the oxyhaemoglobin curve to the left, impairs oxygen delivery to tissues.

Mobilisation of energy resources

Mobilisation of energy resources includes: (a) conversion of liver glycogen to glucose, pyruvate and lactate (a small reserve of only 1600 calories); (b) lysis of proteins: this is 'expensive' (20 cal, 6 g protein) but provides specific amino acid (alanine) for the carbohydrate pathway; and (c) the main source, oxidation of body fat, which can yield 3000 cal/day.

Shock

This is generally defined as circulatory failure, in particular of the microcirculation in tissues. There are several varieties depending on cause, including:

1. *Cardiac*: heart failure (e.g. myocardial infarction)
2. *Neurogenic*: loss of vasomotor tone (e.g. painful stimuli)
3. *Hypovolaemic*: loss of circulating fluid (haemorrhage, other fluid losses)
4. *Endotoxic*: due to bacterial toxins
5. *Anaphylactic*: due to an immune response

Hypovolaemic shock

Typically hypovolaemic shock follows haemorrhage of 20% or more of blood volume, but it may also be associated with the fluid losses of burns and of gut infections such as cholera. The volume deficiency leads to a fall in central venous pressure, reduced venous inflow into the right atrium, a fall in arterial blood pressure, a generalised reduction in tissue perfusion, and tissue hypoxia resulting in a metabolic acidosis. The coronary, brain and adrenal circulations are conserved unless the condition is extreme. The kidney can adapt to moderate falls by decreased vascular resistance. There is a rise in platelets within 1 h and a rise in white cells (mainly polymorphs) within 3–5 h.

Endotoxic shock

Endotoxic shock is caused by the toxins of Gram-negative bacteria, commonly *E. coli*, *Aerobacter aerogenes*, Friedländer's bacillus and *Bacillus proteus*. These toxins are lipocarbohydrates of the bacterial cell wall and act directly on small blood vessels and capillaries. There is also release of cytokines including tumour necrosis factor (TNF). Common sources of infection are septic abortion and any sepsis involving the gut; urinary and biliary infections are less common. Gram-positive organisms can also cause a type of toxic shock (diphtheria and gas gangrene).

The toxic damage to small vessels leads to loss of circulating fluids and proteins into the tissues. The fall in blood volume is thus associated with major fluid and electrolyte disturbances and an increase in blood viscosity (sludging). All of these impair tissue perfusion and cause cell anoxia in every part of the body. The process is often aggravated by disseminated intravascular coagulation due to release of thrombogenic enzymes.

Kidney damage in endotoxic shock is caused by both circulatory changes and direct damage to renal epithelium. The main lesion is necrosis of the proximal convoluted tubules; the process may be reversible after recovery.

Pulmonary complications are common and may be the fatal event. Damage to pulmonary capillaries leads to pulmonary oedema, a rise in vascular resistance and impaired oxygenation of pulmonary blood. The situation is aggravated by patchy atelectasis and opening of arteriovenous shunts, and pneumonitis (staphylococci, *Klebsiella* group) may supervene.

Tumours

A neoplasm has been described as a 'mass of cells which grows at the expense of the organism without serving any useful purpose'. This definition clearly excludes the superficially very similar process of hyperplasia in which normal cells show excessive but appropriate proliferation in response to a specific stimulus.

The rate of growth of tumours is not a defining feature. In most cases it is less than that of the fetus or of some normal cells (e.g. stem cells of bone marrow or intestinal epithelium). If a tumour originates from a single cell and divides regularly, it will take 30 doublings to reach a diameter of 1 cm. Fast-growing tumours (e.g. embryonal sarcoma) have a doubling time of 10–25 days, whereas slow-growing tumours (e.g. cancer of the lip) double in 100 days.

Simple (benign) and malignant tumours

Simple tumours reproduce somewhat the appearance and functions of the cells of origin; they tend to grow slowly and the rate may slow with increasing size; they are often encapsulated. Malignant tumours deviate towards primitive forms and show no growth limitation. Simple tumours grow by expansion and compression of surrounding tissues. Malignant tumours grow by invasion (infiltration) and destruction of other tissues. In addition, they disseminate by metastasis: malignant cells become detached into lymph spaces or blood vessels and thus seed and proliferate in distant sites. There is often only a poor correlation between the size and growth rate of a primary tumour, and the rate and extent of invasion and metastasis.

Tumour histology

Benign tumours are well demarcated from surrounding tissues, whereas most malignant tumours show invasion. Benign tumours repeat the pattern of the tissue of origin, whereas malignant tumours show dedifferentiation and very little architectural pattern. Individual cells of benign tumours may appear entirely normal. Those of malignant tumours show 'anaplasia': they are generally larger than their prototype and of irregular shape; the nucleus is hyperchromatic and vesicular; mitotic figures are common and often of irregular pattern (the number of chromosomes may be decreased or massively increased; abnormal ring-, J- and V-shaped forms may be seen). Dense granules may be seen outside the nucleus and multinucleate giant cells may be present. Of the above features, only invasion is diagnostic. Evidence of anaplasia without apparent invasion is known as carcinoma in situ.

Spread of malignant tumours

1. *Direct invasion* and infiltration of adjacent tissues.

2. *Lymphatic spread*: Commonest in carcinoma, unusual in sarcoma. The spread may occur by direct continuous growth in lymph spaces, reaching successively more distant sites, or, more commonly, by cell embolism, in which clumps of cells are carried to regional lymph nodes to form a secondary deposit.

3. *Haematogenous spread*: Blood-borne metastases are commonest in the 'organs of first encounter' in the venous drainage of the primary tumour: the lungs from the systemic circulation (e.g. kidney, breast, testis, ovary); the liver from the portal circulation (e.g. gut, pancreas), and the bones more directly (e.g. breast, prostate and thyroid). At a later stage there is 'arterial' spread: the liver, adrenals and bone, and to a lesser degree brain and kidneys are involved. The spleen, skeletal muscle, gut, heart, skin and genitourinary organs are rare sites of blood-borne metastasis. Chemotaxis by the endothelial basement membrane protein laminin (but not fibronectin) may explain blood vessel invasion by some tumours.

4. *Implantation of free cells*: Commonest in the peritoneal cavity from adjacent organs, and may also occur as a result of biopsy or surgery.

5. *Spread of cancer from mother to fetus*: Secondary spread of cancer from mother to fetus is rare. The only notable exceptions are melanoma and the lymphoma/leukaemia group.

Incidence of tumours

1. *Age*: There is a general increase with age but striking variations with individual tumours. Sarcoma and lymphomas are common in early life, carcinoma develops later.

2. *Geography*: Examples of geographically related cancers are shown in Table 5.2.

3. *Heredity*: In humans there is clear evidence of tumour inheritance in polyposis coli, neurofibromatosis, albinism, retinoblastoma, phaeochromocytoma and multiple endocrine adenomatosis, and breast cancer. In retinoblastoma there is deletion of a tumour suppressor gene (RB-I) on

Table 5.2. Examples of geographical and racial relationships of cancers

Cancer	Area	Factor
Mouth	India	Betel nut chewing
Bladder	Africa	*Schistosoma haematobium*
Lymphoma (Burkitt's)	Africa	Virus
Nasopharyngeal	China	Virus
Hepatoma	Far East	?
Kaposi's sarcoma	Africa (Zaire)	
Breast (low incidence)	Japan, Singapore, Rumania	
Testis (low incidence)	Negroes	
Oesophagus	China/Southern Africa	
Stomach	Japan	
Choriocarcinoma	West Africa, Far East	

Table 5.3. Examples of cancers related to occupation or other environmental influences. Breakdown products of chemical carcinogens may be as important as the original chemical

Site	Occupation or factor
Bone	Luminous watch painting (radium)
Skin	Paraffin industry
Bladder	Aniline dye industry (notably aromatic amines, 2-naphthylamine)
Bladder	Cyclophosphamide
Lung	Cobalt mining; also chromium and nickel
Mesothelium	Asbestos industry
Scrotum	Chimney sweeps (soot)
Scrotum	Mule spinners (mineral oils)
Lung	Smoking
Gut and bladder	Nitrosamines (foodstuffs)
Skin	Dibenzanthracene and other aromatic hydrocarbons (experimental)
Melanoma	Sunlight (commoner near Equator)
Nasal sinuses	Woodworkers
Liver	Aflatoxins (mould on foods)
Vagina	Stilboestrol treatment of mother in pregnancy

chromosome 11. Early onset breast cancer has been linked to a locus (D17S74) on the long arm of chromosome 17. Conditions in which there is a failure of DNA repair mechanisms have an excess incidence of cancer (xeroderma pigmentosum, ataxia telangiectasia, Fanconi's anaemia).

4. *HLA-types*: women with HLA-DQw3 have a high risk of squamous cell carcinoma of the cervix.

Precancerous states and chemical carcinogens

Some cancers arise from chronic lesions of a non-malignant nature. Examples include congenital anomalies (ectopic testis, neurofibromatosis, polyposis coli) and chronic irritations and ulcers (ulcerative colitis, gall-stones, Bowen's and Paget's diseases of skin). There is also a large group of occupationally and environmentally related cancers (Table 5.3). It should be noted that there is a substantial area of overlap between factors that may be regarded as

Table 5.4. Proto-oncogene abnormalities in human cancer

Cancer	Oncogene abnormality
Burkitt's lymphoma	Translocation of C-myc from chromosome 8 to other chromosomes
Leukaemias	Translocation of C-abl from chromosome 9
Leukaemia	Amplification of C-myc
Colon carcinoma	Amplification of C-myc
Epidermal carcinoma	Amplification of c-erb-B
Neuroblastoma	Amplification of C-myc
Breast carcinoma	Amplification of HER-2/neu on chromosome 17
Colon carcinoma	Mutation of K-ras
Lung adenocarcinoma	Mutation of K-ras
Ovarian carcinoma	Expression of Hα-ras

the cause of precancerous lesions and those that directly cause a cancer (carcinogens).

Viruses as a cause of tumours

Several viruses are associated with tumours in animals, e.g. Rous sarcoma virus (chicken), polyoma virus (mouse leukaemia). Examples of virus associations in human cancer include: hepatoma (hepatitis B), Burkitt's lymphoma (Epstein–Barr virus, which causes translocation of chromosome 14 in lymphocytes), certain nasopharyngeal tumours (Epstein–Barr virus), and carcinoma of the cervix (herpes type II and human papillomavirus). Viruses act by inserting part of their own DNA into the host chromosomes.

Oncogenes

The normal genome contains homologues (C-onc genes or proto-oncogenes) of retroviral transforming genes (V-onc genes). The C-onc genes code for growth factors, which are involved in normal cell proliferation and differentiation. Viral tumorigenesis in animals is caused by V-onc genes. In humans there are two major mechanisms which may convert a normal growth gene into a cancer gene: an alteration in the structure of the gene itself, resulting in an abnormal gene product (somatic mutation); and an increase or decrease in the amount of the gene product, resulting from either gene amplification or changes in control elements. For example, mutant varieties of the tumour suppressor gene p53 can be found in a variety of cancers. Examples of oncogenes in human cancer are shown in Table 5.4. All of the proto-oncogenes are expressed in the human placenta.

Immunity and cancer

There is evidence that the patient's own immune system may play a part in the development of cancer:

1. Some cancers produce tumour-specific transplantation-type antigens.

2. Accumulation of lymphocytes may be seen around the tumour margin.

3. Immune deficiency (e.g. agammaglobulinaemia, treatment with immuno-suppressive agents, AIDS) is associated with a high incidence of reticulo-sarcoma (Kaposi's sarcoma), lymphoma and squamous tumours.

4. Immunotherapy retards the growth of malignant melanoma.

5. Transfusions with blood products, which protect against organ rejection, also promote tumour growth.

In addition, macrophages produce tumour necrosis factor (TNF), which can destroy tumour cells. TNF may be partly responsible for weight loss in advanced cancer.

Tumour products

Certain tumours produce ectopic chemical products. These include:

1. Products not normally produced by the cell of origin (e.g. oat cell carcinoma of the lung may produce ACTH and a wide range of hormones; leiomyosarcoma may produce insulin-like growth factor (IGF) II and thus cause hypoglycaemia). Though comparatively rare, every known hormone has at some time been described as an ectopic product, and virtually every tumour as a producer.

2. Products normally produced by the cell of origin, e.g. carcinoid tumours and 5-hydroxytryptamine; phaeochromocytoma and catecholamines; pancreatic islet cell tumours and gastrin (Zollinger–Ellison syndrome); trophoblast tumours and chorionic gonadotrophin; granulosa cell tumours and inhibin.

3. Products produced by the embryonic equivalent of the cell of origin, e.g. carcinoembryonic antigen and colon cancer; α-fetoprotein and hepatoma.

Tumours from the APUD (amine precursor uptake and decarboxylation) cell system are notable for their secretory characteristics. APUD cells are a group of cells, derived from the neural crest, with a high content of amines (e.g. histamine and dopamine) and polypeptide hormones (e.g. ACTH, insulin, calcitonin and gastrointestinal hormones). They are widely distributed in the gut, pancreatic islets, pituitary and adrenal glands and the parafollicular tissues of the thyroid. Tumours include pituitary adenoma, medullary carcinoma of the thyroid, insulinoma and gastrinoma. Presence of APUD cells may explain other examples of ectopic hormone secretion.

Tumour classification

Hamartomas

These are non-neoplastic but tumour-like congenital malformations. They are present at birth, may grow with the rest of the body but often regress, and are non-invasive. The most familiar type is the angioma, which consists of a network of capillaries and occasional larger blood-filled spaces. The commonest site is the skin (port-wine stain, naevi, telangiectasia); rare sites include the liver, the lung, the bone, the placenta and the nervous system, and occasionally multiple sites (Sturge–Weber syndrome, Lindau's syndrome, Osler–Rendu–Weber syndrome). The glomus tumour (glomangioma) is a specialised arteriovenous anastomosis occurring on the forearm or hand.

Epithelial tumours

Papillomas are benign epithelial tumours projecting from the skin or a mucous membrane (including duct and cyst linings). The skin form is the commonest and includes most warts. Sometimes they are found in the urinary tract and gut; the villous papilloma of the rectum can produce a watery discharge so copious as to cause dehydration and hypokalaemic alkalosis.

Adenomas are benign epithelial tumours of glands. The cells are columnar or pedunculated from a surface (as in familial polyposis coli). If a cyst is formed it is named according to the contents, i.e. serous or mucinous cystadenoma.

Melanomas are tumours of melanocytes. These are neural crest cells, most of which are intercalated into the basal layer of the epidermis. Some but not all contain melanin derived from tyrosine via a colourless intermediate dihydroxyphenylalanine (DOPA). Benign melanomas may be confined to the dermis (naevus cell tumour) or penetrate the epidermis (junctional naevus). Malignant melanomas may arise from a benign lesion (70%) or de novo; the latter may be an early feature and includes unusual sites such as the intestine and the heart. This tumour may metastasise via the placenta to the fetus. The incidence and mortality rates of melanoma are rising, and presentation is occurring at an earlier age. It is commonest in women of reproductive age.

Carcinoma is the commonest malignant tumour, four types occurring:

1. *Squamous cell*: From the skin or the stratified squamous linings of the upper air and food passages and the vagina and cervix, or by metaplasia from the epithelia of the bronchi and urinary tract. Such tumours consist of squamous cells, often arranged in whorls around nests of cornified cells. Sometimes the cells are connected by fibrils (acanthoma or prickle cells). Spread is principally by local invasion and metastasis to regional lymph nodes.

2. *Basal cell* (rodent ulcer): From basal cells of skin, hair follicles and sweat glands, usually on the face around the eyes. These tumours consist of small fusiform cells in masses or columns in a stroma of connective tissue, with no cell nests. Invasion is local and metastasis does not occur.

3. *Glandular carcinoma*: From secretory glands or columnar cell mucous membranes. If gland structure is apparent it is referred to as adenocarcinoma; without such structure, as spheroidal cell carcinoma; and with profuse mucin secretion (giving the cells a 'signet-ring' shape), as mucoid or colloid carcinoma. A mixed squamous and glandular carcinoma occurs in the endometrium and is referred to as adenoacanthoma.

4. *Undifferentiated carcinoma*: This type must be distinguished from lymphoma and amelanotic melanoma by special stains.

Mesenchymal tumours

Fibromas consist of fibroblasts in a stroma of collagen, often arising in relation to nerve sheaths. Multiple fibromas are characteristic of neurofibromatosis. When associated with mucin secretion, fibromas are known as myxomas; when they occur in relation to joints, they are known as synoviomas. Another uncommon type is the infiltrative desmoid tumour occurring in the rectus sheath of parous women.

Lipomas consist of fat cells in a stroma, are usually encapsulated and may occur in any fat tissue, although they are most obvious in subcutaneous tissues. The rare *liposarcoma* is found in the retroperitoneal tissues and may be associated with an unexplained pyrexia.

Myomas are of two types. The leiomyoma occurs in the skin or the gut but the only common form is the uterine fibroid. Rhabdomyomas are rare tumours of striped muscle; they occur in childhood and often become malignant.

Sarcomas are malignant tumours of mesenchyme. They are commonest in childhood and adolescence and may arise from any type of connective tissue (hence the terms fibrosarcoma, chondrosarcoma and osteosarcoma). Sarcomas tend to grow rapidly and metastasise by the bloodstream to the lungs and other sites. Histologically they consist of spindle-shaped or round cells in a stroma, which may indicate the parent tissue. They are highly vascular.

Teratomas

These tumours arise from totipotent cells, which give rise to tissues foreign to the tissue of origin. Most occur in the gonads.

Some characteristics of tumours in special sites

The tumours described here are selected on the basis that they have some functional or anatomical relationship to obstetrics and gynaecology. However, tumours of the female reproductive organs have been excluded as more properly part of a clinical text.

Anterior pituitary

Most tumours of the anterior pituitary are benign adenomas and include: (a) chromophobe adenoma (prolactin or no secretion); (b) craniopharyngioma (no secretion), which occurs in childhood and is sometimes suprasellar; (c) acidophil adenoma (secretes growth hormone); and (d) basophil adenoma (secretes ACTH, Cushing's disease). The first two may cause hypopituitarism via pressure effects.

Phaeochromocytoma

Phaeochromocytoma (usually benign) is derived from chromaffin cells in the adrenal medulla or retroperitoneal tissues and secretes large amounts of catecholamines. The diagnosis is made by measurement of catecholamines in blood or of the excretion product vanillylmandelic acid in urine.

Conn's tumour

Conn's tumour is an adenoma of the adrenal cortex. It secretes aldosterone, causing sodium and water retention and potassium depletion, and thus a hypertensive syndrome.

Carcinoid tumour (argentaffinoma)

Carcinoid tumour is derived from cells that have an affinity for silver stains and which are widely distributed, occurring especially in the intestinal mucosa (Kulchitsky cells). They are slow growing but malignant. The commonest sites are the appendix (60%) and the ileum, and they may occur in ovarian teratoma. Many carcinoids secrete 5-hydroxytryptamine (5-HT) and a spectrum of peptides including tachykinins, but clinical effects (flushing, diarrhoea, bronchospasm, pulmonary stenosis and facial telangiectasia) are rare (occurring in 1% of cases) because the 5-HT is destroyed in the liver. Hormone release can be inhibited by somatostatin.

Bone

The commonest tumour of bone is secondary carcinoma. The commonest sites are the proximal bones: the skull, the spine, the pelvis and the proximal ends of humerus and femur; the bones of the hands and feet are rarely affected. The deposits are usually osteolytic and can be visualised radiologically or by technetium scanning. The effects of osteolysis include breakdown of collagen, with elevated blood levels of hydroxyproline, and calcium release, which may lead to hypercalcaemia.

Breast carcinoma

Breast carcinoma is one of the commonest malignant growths, although only 1% of cases occur in men. The tumour commences in the duct epithelium, most often in the upper outer quadrant. The commonest form is the scirrhous, which is composed of spheroidal epithelial cells in a dense fibrous stroma.

Less common are the atrophic scirrhous, with very few epithelial cells, the medullary, which is bulky, less invasive and has a lymphocytic infiltrate, and adenocarcinoma, which has an acinar structure; all of these have a better prognosis than the scirrhous form.

Breast cancer is rare before the age of 30; thereafter the incidence increases progressively, with a plateau for a few years around the menopause. It is less common in parous than in nulliparous women. The role of hormones in its origin is uncertain, although a wide variety of endocrine manipulations can affect the growth of an established tumour.

Spread by direct invasion may involve both the skin and deep fascia and pectoral muscles. Lymphatic spread is primarily to the axilla (pectoral nodes → central nodes → apical node) and thereafter to the root of the neck and the mediastinum. In some cases the internal mammary nodes are involved, with direct drainage to the mediastinum. Blood-borne metastases may be found in the lungs and bones.

Carcinoma of the colon and rectum

Carcinoma may develop in any part of the colon or rectum. The tumour is a columnar cell adenocarcinoma and may range from totally anaplastic to recognisable gland formation. Local growth is usually annular and constricts the lumen. It may also extend to the mesentery and peritoneum and involve surrounding organs by direct invasion. Lymphatic metastasis is prominent and takes place via local nodes to the para-aortic nodes. Blood-borne metastasis is a late feature and is principally to the liver.

Carcinoma of the bladder

Frequently carcinoma of the bladder arises in apparently benign papillomas, especially those that recur after treatment. The commonest site is the bladder base. Histologically the epithelial cells are of transitional type unless very anaplastic; areas of squamous cells and, very rarely, adenocarcinoma may be seen. Spread is mostly local, through the bladder wall into perivesical tissues. Infiltration of the ureteric orifice and renal failure are common terminal events.

Carcinoma of the prostate

Carcinoma of the prostate is usually an adenocarcinoma with abundant fibrous stroma. Local spread rapidly involves surrounding tissues. Lymphatic spread is to the external and internal iliac nodes. Bone metastases, though a late event, are unusual in that they especially involve the lumbosacral spine, pelvis and femora; this suggests that the origin may be lymphatic rather than blood-borne. Furthermore, they are osteosclerotic rather than osteolytic, a feature attributed to the production of acid phosphatase by the tumour. Measurement of this enzyme in blood is also a useful diagnostic test.

Carcinoma of the prostate is also hormone sensitive, and lengthy remissions can be obtained with oestrogen treatment.

Tumours of the testis

Seminoma arises from spermatocytes and is non-secretory. It constitutes 40% of testicular tumours and is commonest at ages 30–50. Histologically it consists of sheets or columns of polygonal cells with clear cytoplasm and rounded nuclei. It invades and destroys most of the surrounding normal tissues but is usually retained within the tunica albuginea. Spread occurs by lymphatics to the inguinal glands and thence to the para-aortic nodes. Growth is generally slow and prognosis good with early orchidectomy.

Teratomas (30% of testicular tumours) arise from embryonic elements and are commonest at ages 20–45. Histologically they contain a wide variety of ectodermal, mesodermal and endodermal structures, and occasionally (4%) trophoblast (choriocarcinoma). Sometimes the appearance is undifferentiated. They may secrete α-fetoprotein and hCG, which serve as diagnostic and follow-up tests. They are more malignant than seminomas.

Less common tumours include benign dermoid cysts, Sertoli cell tumours and interstitial (Leydig) cell tumours. The latter two (and teratomas) may secrete gonadotrophins and cause gynaecomastia and other features of feminisation.

Thrombosis and embolism

Blood coagulation begins by adhesion of platelets to the vessel wall (particularly exposed collagen) and release of a series of platelet factors including ADP, serotonin, platelet factor 4 and thromboxane A_2 (TXA_2); prostacyclin in the vessel wall has an anti-aggregatory effect. ADP and TXA_2 cause further aggregation of platelets. The coagulation cascade is triggered and leads to formation of an insoluble fibrin clot from circulating fibrinogen (Fig. 5.1). Eventually the platelet mass contracts due to the contractile protein thrombasthenin.

The cascade involves 13 factors (I–XIII) and several subfactors and complexes. Initiation is via an 'intrinsic' pathway (collagen activates factor XII; Hageman factor) or an 'extrinsic' pathway (thromboplastin activates factor VII). The two pathways come together with activation of factor X (Stuart factor), which in turn activates conversion of prothrombin to thrombin. Thrombin further accelerates release of platelet factors.

Specific defects of clotting factors include factor VIII (haemophilia) and factor IX (Christmas disease), both sex-linked recessives. In von Willebrand's disease a factor VIII deficiency (usually dominant) is combined with a vessel wall defect. Vitamin K deficiency due to antagonistic drugs (e.g. coumarin), biliary obstruction or absence of intestinal bacteria (as in haemolytic disease of the newborn) leads to deficiency of factors II, VII, IX and X.

Thrombin splits two small peptides (fibrinogen A and B) from fibrinogen to form fibrin monomer. This then polymerises and in the presence of factor XIII (fibrin stabilising factor) forms the fibrin clot. Normal plasma contains an inhibitor of thrombin (antithrombin III), which acts as a protective mechanism.

The fibrin clot is eventually digested by plasmin. Plasmin is formed from the

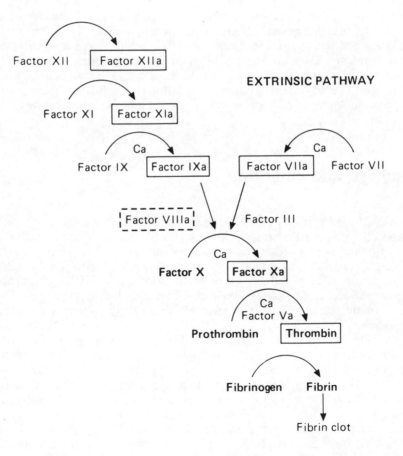

Fig. 5.1. The coagulation cascade. At each step the inactive factor is converted to the active (a) form.

precursor plasminogen in the presence of activators (blood and tissue kinases). Digestion leads to the formation of soluble fibrin degradation products (FDPs, including fragments D and E). FDPs have an anticoagulant effect, interfering with the thrombin–fibrin reaction and with the polymerisation of fibrin, which leads to clot retraction.

Causes of thrombosis

Causes of thrombosis include:

1. Changes in the vessel wall (especially endothelial damage with exposure of underlying collagen)

2. Changes in blood-flow: stasis and eddy-current formation

3. Changes in blood (increase in platelets, polycythaemia vera, hyperlipidaemia, oestrogen therapy)

Atherosclerosis

This is the commonest cause of arterial thrombosis (coronary, cerebral, lower limbs, etc.). It begins as patchy deposits of cholesterol and its esters in the intima at the orifices of arterial branches (eddy sites). The adjacent arterial wall becomes fibrosed and calcified and ulceration may occur. In large vessels mechanical weakening can lead to formation of an aneurysm.

Factors which may be associated with atherosclerosis include hyperlipidaemia (and high fat consumption), generalised diseases such as diabetes, soft water supplies, smoking and obesity.

Deep venous thrombosis

Postoperative thrombosis has an overall incidence of 30% and is commoner in older patients, following operations involving the abdomen and pelvis, following long operations, following operations for malignant disease, and in patients with varicose veins. It usually commences at the time of operation in the veins of the soleus muscle and may spread via the popliteal, femoral and iliac veins to the inferior vena cava. The initial clot consists of fibrin and platelets (a 'white' clot) at a venous valve. Subsequent extension includes many red cells (a 'red' clot).

Pulmonary embolism

The risk of pulmonary embolus is 1% in thrombosis limited to calf muscles, but increases to 50% if the iliofemoral vessels are involved. It usually occurs 1 week or more after operation.

The effects of an embolus include mechanical obstruction of pulmonary vessels and functional obstruction due to release of 5-HT from platelets. A small embolus may have no obvious effect. Larger emboli lead to haemorrhagic infarcts. Massive embolus (60% or more of the pulmonary circulation) causes pulmonary and systemic hypertension, and atelectasis due to decreased concentration of surfactant.

Other forms of embolism

1. *Fat*: after fractures of long bones
2. *Air*: during operation on the head and neck, mismanaged transfusions or haemodialysis, insufflation of fallopian tubes, pneumoperitoneum
3. *Nitrogen*: decompression sickness
4. *Tumour fragments*
5. *Foreign bodies*
6. *Parasites*: *Schistosoma*
7. *Amniotic fluid*: containing meconium and squamous cells

Deposition of salts and pigments

Urinary calculi

Urinary calculi may be formed as a primary result of a metabolic disorder, or secondary to tissue damage and obstruction. They consist of inorganic crystals in a mucoprotein matrix. The inorganic constituent may be: (a) calcium oxalate (the commonest); (b) phosphates of calcium, magnesium and ammonium (infection with *Bacillus proteus* and *Pseudomonas pyocyanea*); (c) uric acid (gout, leukaemia); and (d) cystine (cystinuria) and xanthine (xanthinuria).

Calcium oxalate stones begin in the kidney collecting system and lymphatics of the medulla (nephrocalcinosis). Some 2%–10% of cases are associated with hyperparathyroidism. More commonly, blood calcium is normal but urinary calcium may be raised (50%).

Gall-stones

These consist of varying proportions of cholesterol (the main component), bile salts, bile pigments and calcium salts.

Haemosiderosis and haemochromatosis

Iron overload leads to excessive formation of haemosiderin from haemoglobin. The haemosiderin is deposited in parenchymatous cells of the liver, pancreas, kidney and heart, or in the reticuloendothelial system. Causes include parenteral iron administration, repeated blood transfusions, haemolytic anaemias (especially thalassaemias) and excess dietary iron (Bantu).

A special form is the autosomal recessive condition of haemochromatosis,

Table 5.5. Common forms of ionising radiation

Designation	Nature
Alpha particles (rays)	Helium nucleus (2 protons, 2 neutrons)
Beta particles (rays)	Electrons (negative charge)
Gamma rays	Electromagnetic waves of short wavelength
X-rays	Electromagnetic waves of short wavelength
Protons	Particles (positive charge)
Neutrons	Particles (no charge)

The electromagnetic waves and neutrons have high penetrating power in tissue; other particles have little power.

in which there is excess gut absorption of iron. The organ damage leads to cirrhosis, diabetes mellitus and heart failure.

Effects of radiation

Common forms of ionising radiation are listed in Table 5.5. Passage of radiation through a tissue leads to formation of ions and free radicals and, in high doses (10 000 rads or more), causes immediate death of the cell. Lower doses cause: (a) inhibition of DNA synthesis, (b) delay of mitosis (G_2 phase), (c) abnormal mitosis (chromosome breaks), and (d) slowing of growth. In general, the cells most sensitive to radiation are those of rapid turnover (e.g. bone marrow, intestinal epithelium, cancer cells); neurons and muscle cells are very insensitive. Few tumours divide as rapidly, or are as sensitive, as normal bone marrow and gastrointestinal mucosa, but tumour cells recover more slowly. Repeated doses of radiotherapy therefore deplete tumour cells more effectively than normal cells. Oxygen deficiency reduces sensitivity; metronidazole can restore the sensitivity of hypoxic tissues. The apparent effects of radiation on tissues may be delayed for days or weeks, and the general appearance of irradiated tissues is that of chronic inflammation. Radiation is associated with an increased risk of certain tumours: chronic myeloid leukaemia, squamous cell carcinoma of the skin and osteosarcoma.

Radiotherapy of tumours

Radiotherapy relies for its effect on the production of secondary electrons in tissues, which causes release of energy. The higher the energy of the initial beam, the deeper the area of maximum energy build-up. This fact is used to spare sensitive superficial structures like skin. Radiation energy is measured in rads (1 rad @.004 an energy absorption of 100 ergs per gram of tissue). However, the actual effect on cells varies according to the type of radiation (e.g. neutrons produce 10 times the effect of X-rays). The relative biological efficiency (RBE) is a measure of this. A commonly used unit is the 'roentgen equivalent man' (rem), where dose in rems @.004 rads @.003 RBE.
  Several factors influence the sensitivity of tumours:

1. *Tissue*: Seminomas and lymphoreticular tumours are very sensitive; sarcomas are usually most resistant.

2. *Differentiation*: In general, the less differentiated tumours are the most sensitive.

3. *Tumour bed*: Poorly oxygenated areas (avascular necrosis) are less sensitive. This occurs when the intercapillary distance exceeds 350 μm.

4. *Recurrent tumours*: These tend to be less sensitive than the original tumour.

5. *Tumour type*: Some squamous cell carcinomas are sensitive (skin, cervix); others are not (lung). Adenocarcinomas are generally less sensitive.

Chapter 6

Microbiology

Pathogenic micro-organisms include bacteria, viruses, rickettsiae, myco-plasmas, protozoa and fungi.

Bacteria

Bacteria are single-cell organisms, which may be classified according to both morphology and staining reaction (Table 6.1).

Staphylococcus aureus

Staphylococcus aureus produces a number of enzymes (coagulase, staphy-lokinase and hyaluronidase) and toxins, the latter including an exotoxin which is a common cause of food poisoning and toxic shock syndrome. A number of phage types (I–IV) can be identified. Coagulase-negative staphylococci, known collectively as *Staphylococcus albus*, are skin commensals but may cause catheter-related infections.

The typical lesion produced by *Staph. aureus* is a circumscribed abscess (boils, carbuncles). It can also cause impetigo, pneumonia and toxic shock syndrome.

Streptococci

Streptococci are classified according to their appearance on blood-agar: α-haemolytic (*Strep. viridans*), β-haemolytic and non-haemolytic ('γ-haemolytic'). The β-haemolytic group is further classified into Lancefield groups, of which group A (*Strep. pyogenes*) is the commonest pathogenic organism. *Strep. viridans* and non-haemolytic streptococci (*Strep. faecalis*) are gut commensals.

Table 6.1. Common forms of bacteria

Group	Name	Example	Gram-stain	Features
Cocci	Diplococci	*D. pneumoniae*	+ve	Pairs[c]
	Streptococci	*S. pyogenes*	+ve	Chains[a,b]
	Staphylococci	*S. aureus (pyogenes)*	+ve	Irregular clusters[a,b]
	Neisseria	*N. gonococcus*	−ve	Pairs[c]
	Listeria	*L. monocytogenes*	+ve	
Bacilli	Mycobacterium	*M. tuberculosis*	+ve	Acid-fast by Ziehl–Nielsen[c]
	OBLIGATE AEROBES.			
	Bacillus	*B. anthracis*	+ve	Aerobic, spore-forming
	Clostridium	*Cl. welchii*	+ve	Anaerobic, spore-forming
	Lactobacillus	Döderlein's bacillus	+ve	
	Pseudomonas	*P. pyocyaneus*	−ve	Motile
	Enterobacteriaceae	*E.coli*	−ve	Motile
	Brucella		−ve	
	Bacteroides		−ve	Anaerobic
	Gardnerella	*G.vaginalis*	−ve	
Vibrios		*V. cholera*	−ve	
Spirochetes	Treponema	*T. pallidum*		
	Leptospira	*L. icterohaemorrhagiae*		

[a] Facultative anaerobes.
[b] Non-motile.

Strep. pyogenes produces enzymes (hyaluronidase, streptokinase, DNAase) and haemolysins (streptolysins). Group B streptococci may cause puerperal fever and neonatal meningitis. 'Viridans' streptococci are commensals of the mouth which may cause endocarditis, and *Enterococcus faecalis* ('faecal type streptococcus') are commensals of the gut which may cause urinary tract infections.

The typical lesion produced by *Strep. pyogenes* is spreading cellulitis (including erysipelas and, in combination with other organisms, necrotising fasciitis). It is a common cause of tonsillitis and pharyngitis. If a rash is present this is scarlet fever. Septicaemia occurs readily from ascending genital tract infections (the once-lethal puerperal sepsis). Neonatal septicaemia may occur in the babies of women carrying β-haemolytic streptococci in the vagina. Sequelae to streptococcal infections include rheumatic fever and acute glomerulonephritis.

Gram-negative intestinal bacilli

Most of the organisms causing infections are Enterobacteriaceae, and include *Escherichia*, *Klebsiella* and *Enterobacter*, all of which ferment lactose. *Proteus*, *Shigella* and *Salmonella* (non-lactose fermenters) are also in this group. *Pseudomonas* is a similar but separate group (also non-lactose fermenting).

With the exception of the last three, all these organisms are gut commensals. They contain endotoxin in their cell walls and are opportunistic invaders of tissues. Typical conditions include appendicitis, diverticulitis, ischiorectal abscess, cholecystitis and peritonitis following perforation of the gut. They are the commonest agents in urinary tract infection (*E. coli*) and may be found in postabortal sepsis and pelvic inflammatory disease. Rare sites include the lung (especially *Klebsiella*) and the eye (*Pseudomonas*). Certain strains of *E. coli* can produce an epidemic gastroenteritis, mainly in children. All Gram-negative intestinal organisms can invade the bloodstream and may cause septic shock because of endotoxaemia.

The anaerobic bacteroides form the bulk of organisms in the intestine and are also found in the vagina in 10% of women.

Pneumococcus (*Streptococcus pneumoniae*)

Streptococcus pneumoniae has a very prominent polysaccharide-containing capsule. The most typical lesion is lobar pneumonia, but it can also be involved in otitis media, sinusitis, meningitis, conjunctivitis and a rare primary peritonitis in young girls.

Neisseria

The two pathogenic forms are *N. gonorrhoeae* (gonococcus) and *N. meningitidis* (meningococcus). *N. pharyngitidis* is a commensal of the nasopharynx, as is meningococcus in 10% of normal individuals. The gonococcus will only grow in an atmosphere of 5% carbon dioxide, requires an enriched medium (chocolate agar or Stewart's medium for transport) and is sensitive to cold.

The typical lesion of the gonococcus in males is an acute suppurative urethritis, which rapidly spreads to the accessory glands; the Gram-negative diplococci are seen within the cytoplasm of polymorphs. Other sites include the female urogenital tract, rectum, tonsils and pharynx, and the conjunctiva in newborns. A later complication is monarticular arthritis.

Listeria

Listeria monocytogenes is a Gram-positive rod which is widely distributed in the environment and may be carried in the gut of 1 in 20 people. It can proliferate at low temperature (6°C or above) and high counts may be found on certain soft cheeses, on patés and occasionally on pre-cooked meats. Infection during pregnancy may lead to a flu-like illness or can be asymptomatic; it is sometimes associated with miscarriage, stillbirth and neonatal death.

Clostridia

The most familiar of this group of anaerobes are *Cl. tetani* and *Cl. perfringens*. Their pathogenicity is due to the production of potent exotoxins. *Cl. tetani*

produces a neurotoxin that blocks descending inhibitory fibres in the spinal
cord, causing the rigidity and spasms of tetanus. *Cl. perfringens* produces
a range of enzymes, including lecithinase, which cause severe tissue necrosis (gas gangrene), lymphocytosis and haemolysis. Certain strains of *Cl.
perfringens* are an important cause of food poisoning. The toxin of *Cl.
botulinum* causes a lethal form of food poisoning, botulism.

Tuberculosis

The tubercle bacillus is resistant to stains unless heated (e.g. carbol fuchsin
in the Ziehl–Nielsen method); once stained it resists decolorisation by acid
(acid fast). It grows slowly and only on complex media (Löwenstein–Jensen,
containing glycerol and egg yolk, 6 weeks' culture) but is highly resistant to
drying. The typical lesion is a caseating granuloma known as the tubercle
follicle. It usually begins with a primary focus in the lung and may spread
slowly through lymphatics or rapidly through the bloodstream (miliary tuberculosis). Usually, however, the body overcomes the primary (Ghon) focus and
no further spread occurs. Infection is associated with cell-mediated immunity
as revealed by skin testing with an extract of the organism (purified protein
derivative, 'PPD'; Mantoux and Heaf tests).

Syphilis

Treponema pallidum is a spiral filament which can only be visualised by
dark-ground illumination or fluorescent-antibody techniques, and does not
grow in culture. Infection is associated with development of two groups of
antibodies:

1. *Reagin (Wasserman) antibody*: Directed towards phospholipids (cardio-
lipin) and the basis of the Wasserman test (complement fixation) and the
Kahn and VDRL tests (flocculation). The antigen is not specific, and a
positive reaction may be found in a variety of other chronic infections, in
collagenoses and in pregnancy.

2. *Treponemal group antibody*: Specific to treponemal proteins. Tests
become positive 1–3 weeks after primary infection and include Reiter's protein complement fixation (RPCF), *Treponema pallidum* haemagglutination
(TPHA), *Treponema pallidum* immobilisation (TPI) and fluorescent treponemal antibody (FTA). With the exception of TPI, these tests are not
specific for the pallidum species (e.g. positive TPHA in yaws, *Tr. pertenue*).
They detect IgG antibodies and therefore results may remain positive for
many years after treatment, unlike those of the reagin tests (e.g. VDRL),
which may be used to monitor the effects of treatment.

Treponema pallidum is very sensitive to both water and drying; hence the
infection occurs only by intimate venereal contact. It is highly invasive and
spreads very rapidly via lymphatics and the bloodstream. It may cross the
placenta after the 16th week of pregnancy.

Table 6.2. A classification of viruses

RNA-containing viruses	
Picornaviruses	Enteroviruses (Coxsackie, ECHO, polio) and rhinoviruses (common cold)
Reoviruses (including rotaviruses)	Respiratory tract infections and diarrhoea in in children
Myxoviruses	Influenza
Paramyxoviruses	Mumps, para-influenza, measles, respiratory syncytial virus
Arboviruses (arthropod borne)	Encephalitis, yellow fever, dengue, sandfly fever
Rhabdoviruses	Rabies
Retroviruses	HIV, HTLV-1
DNA-containing viruses	
Adenoviruses	Respiratory tract infections, keratoconjunctivitis
Papovaviruses	Verrucae
Herpesviruses	Herpes simplex, varicella-zoster, cytomegalovirus, infectious mononucleosis (Epstein–Barr virus), HHV-6
Poxviruses	Smallpox, vaccinia, molluscum contagiosum
Hepadnaviruses	Hepatitis B

Actinomycosis

Actinomyces are anaerobic Gram-positive branching filaments, which tend to grow as a dense mass with a fringe of club-shaped excrescences ('sulphur granules' in pus). The human form, *Actinomyces israeli,* is a mouth commensal which, following trauma, may form chronic suppurative foci in the lower jaw. It is a rare cause of unilateral salpingitis and is more likely to occur in women who have an intrauterine device.

Viruses

These are the smallest of infectious agents and, with the exception of pox viruses, can only be visualised by electron microscopy. They consist of a core of nucleic acid (DNA or RNA) with a protein shell (capsid) arranged as identical subunits (capsomeres). The proteins may include enzymes, but never the full range required for independent existence: hence viruses are obligatory intracellular parasites. A classification of viruses is shown in Table 6.2.

The process of cell infection by a virus includes:

1. Attachment to surface receptors

2. Penetration of the membrane

3. An eclipse phase during which the virus usually redirects cell metabolism (and is non-infective)

4. A phase of maturation and replication during which clumps of virus visible by light microscopy may be formed (visible as inclusion bodies, e.g. in cytomegalovirus, herpes, rabies (the Negri body))

5. A phase of release, which may be rapid (poliovirus) or a steady leakage (HIV, myxoviruses): once released, the virus can attack other cells

Because of their characteristics, viruses can be grown only in intact cells: (a) in whole animals (e.g. suckling mice, chick embryos), (b) in cultured cells (e.g. monkey kidney cells, human amnion and strains of cancer cells such as HeLa) or (c) in organ cultures (e.g. trachea).

Viruses produce disease by causing cell destruction followed by an inflammatory ... on factors ... bacterial toxins. The immun...

1. I... ...lood during ... ...olio, measl... ...cous memb... ...vent attach...

2. I... ...limination ... ...bulin defici...

3. ...

Be... ...mple cultur... ...ically (i.e. ... ...s are becom... ...ctron micr...

[Handwritten note on card:]
PHYSICALLY HANDICAPPED FOLKS DIED CYCLING
HEP A — PICONAVIRUS
HEP B — HEPADNAN VIRUS ✱
HEP C — FLAVIVIRUS
HEP D — DEFECTIVE VIRUS
HEP E — CALCI VIRUS
✱ B is only DNA virus

COVERSYL PLUS   COVERSYL

Some common viral diseases

Enterovirus infections

These include infections by Coxsackie virus, ECHO virus and polioviruses. They are typically found in the gut and faeces, and spread as epidemics. They cause a wide spectrum of disease including pyrexia of unknown origin, aseptic meningitis and, in the case of poliovirus, paralysis. Poliomyelitis (incubation period 7–14 days) enters the blood via the bowel lymphatics. Infection is often subclinical, but may localise in the anterior horn cells and cause widespread paralysis. Active immunisation was originally achieved with the use of formol-inactivated virus grown in monkey kidney cells. Subsequently this was replaced by the use of attenuated strains of poliovirus (Sabin), which do not invade the CNS and are given orally.

Respiratory virus infection

Numerous viruses may infect the upper respiratory tract. Influenza occurs in types A, B and C. Influenza A is responsible for major epidemics (e.g. Asian 'flu); the appearance of new strains preempts immunity due to previous infections. Influenza B is endemic and causes circumscribed outbreaks. The adenoviruses are frequent causes of childhood infections, often associated with conjunctivitis. The rhinoviruses are responsible for the common cold.

Virus hepatitis

There are at least five types of 'infectious' hepatitis: A, B, C, D and E. In addition, other viral agents such as infectious mononucleosis and cytomegalovirus can cause hepatitis as part of a more generalised infection. Infective hepatitis (virus A, picornavirus, incubation 15–40 days) occurs epidemically in institutions and in developing countries; the virus is excreted in faeces (in which it can be detected by an immunoassay) and spread by contaminated food and water. There is no carrier state. Hepatitis B (virus B, DNA, incubation 60–160 days) is usually transmitted by inoculation of blood products (e.g. transfusion, contaminated needles shared by drug addicts) or by close person-to-person contact such as between mother and baby. Persons handling blood or working in haemodialysis units are therefore at special risk. Hepatitis A and B may both be sexually transmitted.

Three antigens are associated with hepatitis B infection:

1. *HBsAg*: The outer coat of the virus (visualised by electron microscopy as the Dane particle) has a surface antigen (HBsAg, originally known as Australia antigen), which is always present in the acute phase of infection and also in the chronic carrier. The appearance of antibody to HBsAg indicates recovery and subsequent immunity.

2. *HBcAg*: This is the core antigen, which is not detected in serum. IgM antibodies to HBcAg appear during acute infection and IgG antibodies indicate past exposure.

3. *HBeAg*: This antigen is associated with infectivity. It is detectable in serum during acute infection and in carriers with a high risk of transmission. Antibodies to HBeAg indicate a low risk of transmission.

Many patients who have been infected with hepatitis B virus, either overtly or subclinically, continue to excrete the virus (carrier rates range from 0.1% in the UK to 15% in the Far East and Africa). HBsAg carriers who continue to express e-antigen are considered to be more infectious than others, and to have a higher risk of chronic liver disease and hepatoma. HBsAg-positive mothers with the e-antigen or lacking anti-e antibodies may infect their infants after delivery. In acute cases the virus can cross the placenta. Thus, acute infection with hepatitis B may be transmitted to the fetus, especially in the third trimester, and cause stillbirth or neonatal hepatitis. Passive immunisation with immunoglobulins containing anti-HBs antibodies is indicated for babies of e-antigen-positive mothers and those with HBsAg but no anti-e antibodies. This will prevent these infants from becoming carriers. Passive immunisation should be followed by active immunisation with hepatitis B vaccine.

Herpes virus infections

These DNA viruses include varicella-zoster, herpes simplex (HSV-1 and HSV-2), cytomegalovirus, Epstein–Barr and HHV-6.

Herpes simplex type 1 can cause superficial lesions of the face, mouth, pharynx and cornea. Severe generalised HSV-1 infection can occur in the neonate, where it is frequently associated with encephalitis and has a mortality rate of 90% if untreated. The virus can remain latent in the trigeminal ganglion

Table 6.3. Acquisition of perinatal viral infection

Virus	Transplacental spread	Infection from latent or current disease	Perinatal infection in the presence of maternal antibodies
Rubella	+ + +	−	−
Hepatitis B	+	+	Rarely, possibly never
Cytomegalovirus	+ +	+	+
Herpes simplex	Very rare	+	+

and other sites. Herpes simplex type 2 is transmitted sexually or intrapartum. Primary infections may be associated with a benign aseptic meningitis or a sacral radiculitis. The genital lesions may be recurrent; the virus has long quiescent stages in sacral ganglia from which it re-infects the epithelial surfaces. Very rarely both HSV-1 and HSV-2 can cause severe neonatal infections: infection may occur even in the presence of maternal antibody (Table 6.3).

Cytomegalovirus is transmitted across the placenta and can cause a lethal infection in neonates; the parenchymatous cells of many organs are distended with large intranuclear inclusion bodies, which may also be found in urine of infected infants. This condition occurs in less than 1 in 10 000 newborns in the UK. Maternal antibody does not prevent perinatal infection (Table 6.3).

The Epstein–Barr virus is associated with Burkitt's lymphoma, naso-pharyngeal carcinoma and infectious mononucleosis.

Rubella (German measles)   CRNA)

Rubella is a trivial infection, but if it occurs in the first 4 months of pregnancy there is a high incidence of congenital abnormalities (up to 4 weeks, more than 60%; 4–8 weeks 25%; 8–12 weeks 10%; 12–16 weeks 5%). The abnormalities include heart lesions, cataracts and deafness; mental deficiency is uncommon. Recent maternal infection can be diagnosed by a rising antibody titre or the appearance of specific IgM antibodies. The latter appear at the time of onset of the rash and become undetectable within 2–3 months. The incubation period is 14–21 days. Recurrent infection is possible and causes a rise in antibody titre, but viraemia and transplacental spread occur rarely. Prevention is achieved through routine vaccination (age 18 months) with attenuated measles–mumps–rubella vaccine (MMR). Congenital infection is a theoretical possibility with this vaccine and it should not be administered during pregnancy.

Human parvovirus

Maternal infection (rubella-like rash, arthritis) can lead to mid-trimester abortion with gross hydrops and anaemia of the fetus.

Acquired immune deficiency syndrome (AIDS)

This syndrome is caused by infection with human immunodeficiency virus (HIV). This is a retrovirus, which contains reverse transcriptase, and thus can manufacture DNA from the original RNA. This DNA becomes incorporated in the host genome, where it codes for the formation of new virus. HIV recognises the CD4 receptor molecule on T-helper cells and thus gains entry to the cell. Even incomplete virus can recognise this receptor, and combination of the protein coat of HIV with the CD4 molecule can cause fusion and ultimately destruction of T-helper cells, thus aggravating the pathology of the disease.

HIV is transmitted by body fluids (including blood, breast milk, vaginal secretions and seminal fluid) and by sexual intercourse in particular. AIDS is a sexually transmitted disease which can also be transmitted by blood products (transfusion, factor VIII, drug abuse) and from mother to baby. HIV can be transmitted by artificial insemination. It is associated with opportunistic infection and a high incidence of Kaposi's sarcoma and lymphomata. Of those with clinical AIDS, few survive more than 2 years and the case fatality rate is probably 100%. Antibodies to HIV usually appear by 3 months after infection. The presence of antibodies is associated with presence of the virus, i.e. seropositive people should be regarded as infectious. At least 80% of infected subjects develop clinical disease. If untreated, the mean incubation period is 52 months. Seropositive women have about a 30% risk of passing HIV to the fetus, which may develop clinical AIDS after birth.

Human papillomavirus

Human papillomavirus (HPV) is a DNA virus with numerous subtypes, which infects the basal cells of squamous epithelia and causes proliferative lesions, the commonest being simple skin warts. Subtypes 6 and 11 are associated with benign genital warts and low grades of cervical intraepithelial neoplasia (CIN); HPV 16 and 18 are associated with most CIN lesions of all grades and invasive cancer. In CIN the virus is free in the cell; in malignant cells the DNA is integrated into various chromosomes. Some 30% of women with vulval condylomata acuminata develop CIN. HPV has been detected in 90% of cervical carcinomas.

Rickettsial organisms

Rickettsia contain DNA and RNA and are therefore similar to bacteria. They have a cell wall and divide by binary fission, but cannot create their own energy and are unable to grow in cell-free media. They are generally sensitive to tetracyclines and erythromycin.

The main genera are *Rickettsia* (typhus and typhus-like fevers transmitted by arthropods), *Coxiella* (Q-fever), *Bartonella* (Oroya fever) and *Chlamydia* (psittacosis, lymphogranuloma venereum, trachoma and genital infections).

Chlamydia trachomatis causes urethritis (50% of cases of non-gonococcal urethritis), salpingitis, cervicitis and epididymitis, and is responsible for a neonatal pneumonia syndrome and late-onset neonatal conjunctivitis. Chlamydial salpingitis may be associated with peritonitis and perihepatitis (Fitz-High–Curtis syndrome).

Mycoplasmas (pleuropneumonia-like organisms)

Mycoplasmas are Gram-negative bacteria lacking a cell wall. The best known is *Mycoplasma pneumoniae* (Eaton agent). Other strains (*Ureaplasma urealyticum*) are found in the mouth and genital tract and may be involved in non-gonococcal urethritis.

Fungal infections

Pathogenic fungal infections include blastomycosis, cryptococcosis, histoplasmosis and coccidioidomycosis: these are caused by dimorphic fungi present in soil, which are yeast-like at body temperature and mould-like at room temperature. They may produce pulmonary lesions when inhaled by immunocompetent subjects. Cryptococcosis may cause meningitis in immunocompromised subjects.

Candidiasis is far commoner. *Candida* is a Gram-positive yeast, which reproduces by budding and is a commensal in the mouth, gut and vagina. *Candida albicans* is the commonest species but 10% of infections are due to *C. glabrata*. Growth is selected for in acid conditions (Sabouraud's medium). It causes superficial infections on mucous membranes (thrush). The vaginal and vulval infection is common in pregnancy and in diabetes mellitus; in both there is an excess of glycogen in vaginal cells, which is fermented by the yeast. In conditions of deficient cell-mediated immunity (e.g. following administration of cytotoxic drugs) a severe systemic infection may occur.

Protozoal infections

These include malaria, leishmaniasis, trypanosomiasis, amoebiasis, toxoplasmosis and pneumocystis pneumoniae.

Toxoplasma gondii is spread by cats. Serological evidence of previous infection is present in 33%–90% of humans and may be reactivated in immunodeficiency states such as AIDS and organ transplants. In adults it may cause a febrile illness but is usually asymptomatic. The fetus is infected only when the mother acquires a primary infection during or shortly before pregnancy, when 50% will be affected (incidence estimated to be from 1 in 1000 to 1 in 8000 live births). This can lead to abortion, stillbirth or neonatal infection. Cerebral calcification is an important feature of the latter, together with retinitis (blindness), hepatitis, microcephaly and thrombocytopenia. The acute infection in pregnancy can be treated with spiramycin if the fetus is not infected, or sulphadiazine and pyrimethamine if it is infected.

Trichomonas organisms may exist as commensals in the gut. Both *Trich. hominis* (gut) and *Trich. vaginalis* (vagina) are pear-shaped with three to five flagella at the broad front end and another flagellum forming part of an undulating membrane at the posterior end. *Trichomonas* survives well in ordinary water, even when this is hot or contains chlorine or detergents. In the presence of a trichomonal infection the normal rod-shaped lactobacilli of the vagina adopt a round, coccoidal form.

Some characteristics of infections at special sites

Wound infection

The commonest organism is *Staph. aureus*. Group A streptococcal infection is now infrequent but dangerous. In wounds related to the gut, *E. coli* may be involved. Special types of anaerobic wound infection include *Cl. perfringens* (amputations) and bacteroides (abdominal wounds). *Cl. tetani* infections of penetrating wounds may lead to tetanus in the non-immunized.

Urinary infections

These are usually caused by Gram-negative intestinal bacilli, the commonest being *E. coli*. Infections with other Enterobacteriaceae and *Pseudomonas* may be the result of cross-infection due to catheterisation and bladder drainage. *Proteus* infection causes urine to become alkaline and, if recurrent, may lead to stone formation.

Food poisoning

Diseases transmitted by food or water include typhoid fever, bacillary dysentery (*Shigella*), amoebiasis, poliomyelitis and hepatitis A. The classical form of simple 'food poisoning', i.e. acute gastroenteritis, may be caused by: (a) *Salmonella* (e.g. *S. enteritidis*, incubation 12–24 h); (b) staphylococcal enterotoxins (incubation 1–6 h); (c) *Cl. perfringens* (incubation 2–24 h, common in the elderly); (d) norwalk agent (the cause of winter vomiting disease) and rotavirus (an important cause of dehydrating enteritis in children); (e) *Campylobacter* (acquired from cooked poultry and contaminated milk); and (f) *Bacillus cereus* (acquired from pre-cooked rice).

All of these conditions are caused by either inadequately cooked food, or cooked food which has been contaminated and then stored at a temperature that allows proliferation of the organisms.

Chapter 7

Pharmacology

The drugs described here are those typically encountered in the current practice of obstetrics and gynaecology. Highly specialised applications have been omitted, as have agents which are largely of historical interest (e.g. most barbiturates).

Sedative, hypnotic and anxiolytic agents

The three actions of sedation, sleep induction (hypnotic action) and reduction of anxiety are very closely related: all drugs in this class will have, in some degree, all three effects. In current practice, virtually all agents of this type are benzodiazepines (Table 7.1), and the use of materials such as paraldehyde, chloral hydrate and barbiturates for these indications is now of only historical interest. Features common to all benzodiazepines include the following:

1. They all cross the placenta (umbilical blood levels 40%–70% of maternal) and should be avoided in late pregnancy other than for specific indications.

2. Their effects are potentiated by alcohol.

3. They are addictive, and withdrawal following long-term use should be gradual.

4. In late pregnancy short-acting agents are preferable (oxazepam, temazepam).

Antipsychotic agents

These are also termed neuroleptics; they tranquillise without impairing consciousness and also have anti-emetic effects. The main action is blocking of dopamine receptors, hence the two notable side-effects of hyperpro-lactinaemia (and thus disturbances of ovulation and menstruation) and

Table 7.1.   Examples of commonly used benzodiazepines

Agent	Features
Long-acting hypnotics	
Nitrazepam (Mogadon)	Used for early morning insomnia but may cause hangover
Flurazepam (Dalmane)	As nitrazepam
Short-acting hypnotics	
Temazepam (Euhypnos)	Hypnotic, shorter-acting than nitrazepam
Triazolam (Halcion)	As temazepam
Anxiolytics	
Diazepam (Valium)	
Chlordiazepoxide (Librium)	
Clorazepate (Tranxene)	
Lorazepam (Ativan)	

Table 7.2.   Major groups of antipsychotic agents

Phenothiazines	
Group 1 (chlorpromazine)	Pronounced sedative effects; moderate anticholinergic and extrapyramidal effects
Group 2 (pericyazine, thioridazine)	Moderately sedative, marked anticholinergic but minimal extrapyramidal effects
Group 3 (fluphenazine, perphenazine, prochlorperazine)	Minimal sedative and anticholinergic effects; pronounced extrapyramidal effects
Butyrophenones	
Haloperidol, pimozide	Resemble group 3 phenothiazines
Thioxanthenes	
Chlorprothixene, flupenthixol	Resemble group 3 phenothiazines

extrapyramidal disturbances (dystonia and a Parkinson-like syndrome). They also have anticholinergic effects (dry mouth, constipation, difficulty with micturition, blurring of vision). Other side-effects include hypothermia, weight gain and cholestatic jaundice. The main group of antipsychotics are shown in Table 7.2. They all cross the placenta.

A very distinct group of these agents is the lithium salts. These are used only for manic depressive psychosis and can be highly toxic, causing polyuria and, in high doses, encephalopathy.

Antidepressive agents

The two main groups are the tricyclic and tetracyclic antidepressants and monoamine oxidase inhibitors (MAOI). The tricyclics prevent noradrenaline re-uptake by nerve cells and can be divided into those which have marked sedative effects (e.g. amitriptyline) and those which are less sedative (e.g. imipramine). The main side-effects are anticholinergic effects and cardiac arrhythmias and heart block. They also interfere with some antihypertensive drugs (ganglion blockers).

The MAOI (e.g. phenelzine, iproniazid) may greatly potentiate the pressor effect of tyramine present in certain foods (cheese, pickled herring, broad bean pods, meat and yeast extracts and Chianti wine). They also have unfavourable interactions with many other drugs – notably the sympathomimetic agents present in many cough mixtures.

Another important group is the serotonin uptake inhibitors (e.g. fluoxetine (Prozac), paroxetine). These have fewer side effects than the tricyclics.

Analgesics

The non-narcotic analgesics include aspirin, paracetamol and a series of newer agents (e.g. fenoprofen, flufenamic acid, mefenamic acid, naproxen). The latter are broadly similar to aspirin in both their effects and side-effects, but tend to be used for their antipyretic, anti-inflammatory (arthritis) or antiprostaglandin (dysmenorrhoea) properties. The major side-effects of aspirin are gastrointestinal irritation and haemorrhage and, in large doses, tinnitus. Aspirin, like other acid drugs, is more ionised in alkaline solution. As the ionised fraction cannot be reabsorbed by the tubule, renal excretion is potentiated by alkalinising the urine. Aspirin is not teratogenic. The main side-effects of paracetamol are renal and hepatic damage (on very large and prolonged dosage).

The narcotic analgesics are, in approximate order of potency: dextropropoxyphene, codeine, dihydrocodeine, pentazocine, pethidine, phenazocine, methadone, morphine and diamorphine (heroin). They all have in common that they may cause (albeit in relatively differing degrees) constipation, respiratory depression, cough suppression, urinary retention, nausea, tolerance and addiction. Some features of individual agents are shown in Table 7.3. All drugs of this class act via specific membrane receptors in brain cells; these 'opiate' receptors are identical with those of the naturally occurring endorphins (peptides of the ACTH-LPH family). They cross the placenta

Table 7.3. Features of some narcotic analgesic agents

Agent	Feature
Codeine, dihydrocodeine	Used for moderate pain; can cause dizziness and constipation
Pentazocine	Can cause hallucinations and rise in blood pressure (avoid in myocardial infarction)
Pethidine	Used in labour and for pain associated with intracranial damage. Short-acting and causes less respiratory depression than other agents
Meptazinol	Similar effects to pethidine but causes less respiratory depression in neonate
Phenazocine	Used in biliary colic (less tendency to raise biliary pressure than other agents)
Morphine	Commonly used for severe pain; produces euphoria and mental detachment
Diamorphine	Very potent; causes less nausea and constipation than morphine

Table 7.4. Features of antacid agents

Agent	Features
Insoluble salts of aluminium and magnesium	Long acting; magnesium salts can cause diarrhoea
Sodium bicarbonate	Short-acting; excessive use can cause alkalosis
Dimethicone	Anti-foaming agent
Alginates	Provide protective coating for mucosa
Calcium salts	May *increase* gastric acidity; constipation
Bismuth salts	Weak. Can cause encephalopathy
Local anaesthetics (oxethazaine)	
Carbenoxolone	Anti-ulcer agent (mainly gastric). Can cause hypernatraemia and hypokalaemia and aggravates hypertension
Cimetidine	Anti-ulcer agent (mainly duodenal). Blocks H_2-receptors and reduces acid secretion. Causes gynaecomastia in men due to inhibition of metabolism of oestradiol

Table 7.5. Features of commonly used laxatives

Agent	Features
Bulk-forming agents (bran, ispaghula husk, methylcellulose, sterculia)	Can cause obstruction
Mild intestinal stimulants (bisacodyl, phenolphthalein, senna, cascara, castor oil)	Can cause atonic colon and hypokalaemia with prolonged use
Parasympathomimetic stimulants (bethanecol, neostigmine)	Used for paralytic ileus and postoperative urinary retention
Faecal softeners (liquid paraffin, dioctyl sodium sulphosuccinate)	Used for haemorrhoids and anal fissure
Osmotic laxatives (lactulose, magnesium salts)	

readily and levels in umbilical blood are 60%–100% of those in the mother. The effects of narcotic analgesics (e.g. severe respiratory depression and coma) can be reversed by naloxone (Narcan).

Antacids

Features of antacids are shown in Table 7.4. Only the insoluble salts of magnesium and aluminium should be used in pregnancy.

Laxatives

Features of laxatives are shown in Table 7.5.

Anti-emetics

The most effective agents are atropine and hyoscine, but these have very pronounced anticholinergic side-effects. For morning sickness either phenothiazine derivatives (e.g. promethazine) or antihistamines (e.g. dimenhydrinate) may be used if felt to be essential, although these may also cause moderate drowsiness and anticholinergic effects. Metoclopramide is particularly useful before anaesthesia because it combines a central phenothiazine-like effect with gastric emptying.

Antihistamines

Histamine acts through H_1-receptors (causing smooth muscle contraction in the intestine, bronchioles, uterus and large blood vessels, and dilatation of small vessels leading to hypotension and headache) and H_2-receptors (stimulating gastric acid secretion). H_1-antagonists include chlorpheniramine, and newer agents such as terfenadine which are less sedative. H_2-antagonists include cimetidine (Tagamet) and ramitidine (Zantac), which may cause gynaecomastia, galactorrhoea and mental confusion.

Diuretics

The characteristics of the most familiar groups of diuretics are listed in Table 7.6. Thiazides have been widely used in treatment of pre-eclampsia, but as this condition is already associated with a decreased plasma volume they may further diminish placental blood-flow and should be avoided. Furthermore, they may cause neonatal thrombocytopenia.

Antihypertensive agents

The maintenance of normal blood pressure depends on a variety of inter-related factors, including the extracellular fluid volume (salt and water metabolism), the cardiac output, the autonomic nerve supply to vessels and the renin–angiotensin–aldosterone system. Any or all of these may be involved in hypertension (including pre-eclampsia) and provide targets

Table 7.6. Features of commonly used diuretics

Agent	Mechanism	Features
Thiazides (bendrofluazide, chlorothiazide, chlorthalidone)	Inhibit Na^+ and K^+ absorption at beginning of proximal convoluted tubule	Can cause hypokalaemia, hypochloraemic alkalosis, hyperuricaemia and hyperglycaemia
Loop diuretics (frusemide, ethacrynic acid)	Inhibit Na^+ and K^+ absorption in ascending loop of Henle	More potent than thiazides (including side-effects); pancreatitis
Potassium-sparing diuretics (amiloride, triamterene)		Weak diuretics, but conserve potassium
Spironolactone	Antagonises aldosterone	Causes potassium retention; used in primary and secondary hyper-aldosteronism
Osmotic diuretics (mannitol, urea)	Expand blood volume	May be useful in cerebral oedema
Mercurial diuretics (mersalyl)		Nephrotoxic

for specific therapy for the lowering of blood pressure. The properties of commonly used agents are summarised in Table 7.7.

Drugs affecting blood coagulation

Anticoagulants

Heparin

Heparin is a high molecular weight (8000–17 000) polysaccharide extracted from mammalian lung and liver, where it is stored in mast cells. Its action results from the strong anionic activity of sulphate groups and is neutralised by compounds with cationic groups (e.g. protamine). Heparin does not pass the placental barrier and is not secreted into urine or milk.

In addition to its anticoagulant effect in vitro and in vivo, heparin activates lipoprotein lipase and thus clears lipaemic plasma. The principal effect on clotting is inhibition of the conversion of fibrinogen to fibrin by thrombin. This action normally requires the presence of heparin cofactor (antithrombin III). Heparin also inhibits activated factor X (Xa). The dosage of heparin can be monitored by its effect on whole blood clotting time or by measurement of factor Xa activity.

Side-effects of heparin therapy include haemorrhage, hypersensitivity reactions, occasionally thrombocytopenia, and osteoporosis after prolonged administration.

Coumarins and indanediones

Coumarins and indanediones are active only in vivo. They are absorbed from the gut and interfere with the hepatic synthesis of factors II (prothrombin),

Table 7.7. Antihypertensive agents[a]

Agent	Mechanism	Features
β-Adrenergic blockers (propranolol, oxprenolol, atenolol, labetalol (α and β))	Reduction of cardiac output, inhibition of renin release, peripheral effect on adrenergic receptors	Slow acting (hours to days) May cause growth retardation if given early in pregnancy
α-Adrenergic blockers (phentolamine, phenoxy-benzamine)		Only used in cases of excess catecholamine secretion
Centrally acting drugs (methyldopa, clonidine)	Act on α-receptors in brainstem to reduce sympathetic activity	Slow acting, can cause sedation, depression and autoimmune anaemia (methyldopa)
Noradrenaline-depleting agents (reserpine)		Can cause severe depression
Vasodilators (hydralazine, diazoxide)	Direct action on walls of arterioles	Fast acting Hydralazine can cause a lupus syndrome Diazoxide can cause water retention and hyperglycaemia
Adrenergic ganglion blockers (guanethidine)	Prevent release of noradrenaline from adrenergic nerve endings (both α- and β-responses)	Cause severe postural hypotension
ACE inhibitors (captopril, enalapril)	Prevents conversion of angiotensin I to angiotensin II; very effective in combination with diuretics	First dose should be given in hospital Causes fetal death
Calcium antagonists (nifedipine, verapamil)	Inhibit entry of calcium into cells	May cause throbbing headache Relax the uterus
Ketanserin	Blocks serotonin (5-HT) receptors	

[a] Diuretics are considered elsewhere. Note that all agents can cause postural hypotension, but this is especially severe with the adrenergic blockers.

VII, IX and X by competing with the action of vitamin K. The action has a latent period of 12–24 h; a large loading dose is followed by a maintenance dose monitored according to the prothrombin time, which reflects primarily a combination of factors VII and X. The most important indanedione is phenindione, and the most widely used coumarin is warfarin. These drugs cause a rapid decrease of factors VII and IX (which have short half-lives of 12 h), and a slower decrease of factor X (half-life 3 days).

Adverse effects other than haemorrhage include alopecia, urticaria and gangrenous skin rashes. All of these drugs cross the placenta and may cause chondrodysplasia punctata and facial bone abnormalities in the first-trimester fetus and haemorrhagic disease of the newborn when administered near term. They are secreted in breast milk (phenindione more so than warfarin). Many drugs (e.g. phenylbutazone) compete with coumarins for binding sites on albumin and hence enhance their anticoagulant effect. Broad-spectrum antibiotics potentiate the action by decreasing endogenous intestinal vitamin K formation. Barbiturates increase coumarin catabolism in the liver.

Vitamin K is the most effective antagonist of these drugs, but acts after a latent period of 8 h and produces its maximal effect after 1 day. For a rapid reversal, fresh-frozen plasma must be used.

Activators of the fibrinolytic system

Certain strains of haemolytic streptococci produce an enzyme, streptokinase, which converts inactive plasminogen into plasmin. Streptokinase is active only when given parenterally. It is highly allergenic, and repeated administration carries the risk of immediate and delayed hypersensitivity reactions.

Most tissues contain plasminogen activators. One of these (urokinase) can be concentrated from human urine. It is non-allergenic but contains a small amount of undesirable thromboplastin activity. A tissue plasminogen activator (TPA) is produced by recombinant DNA technology.

Antifibrinolytics

1. *ε-Aminocaproic acid (EACA)*: This competes with plasminogen activator, thus preventing the formation of plasmin. It is active orally or systemically. Side-effects include risk of thrombosis due to complete blockage of fibrinolytic activity. It can also produce clot retention (e.g. in the ureter in haematuria).

2. *Tranexamic acid*: This is more potent than EACA and has a similar action.

3. *Aprotinin (Trasylol)*: This polypeptide is prepared from bovine lung and is a potent protease inhibitor when given systemically. It is effective against plasmin *and* plasminogen activators and also blocks the formation of thromboplastin. Thus, unlike EACA, it controls both hyperplasminaemic and hypercoagulable states and is less likely to induce thrombosis. It also inactivates kallikrein and trypsin.

Antiplatelet drugs

These include dipyridamole, aspirin and sulphinpyrazone. The last two act as platelet cyclo-oxygenase inhibitors, thus preventing formation of endoperoxides and thromboxane.

Drugs used for treatment of osteoporosis

Oestrogen treatment is widely employed in postmenopausal women for prevention of osteoporosis. Many other drugs have been investigated, including fluoride, calcitonin and biphosphonates. The latter inhibit osteoclast-mediated bone resorption and lead to increased bone mass and a decreased fracture rate.

Chemotherapy of infection

Antibiotics

The most important groups of antibiotics are listed in Table 7.8. The penicillins and cephalosporins attack bacterial cell walls; for this reason they have little effect on host metabolism and few side-effects. All antibiotics may cause allergic reactions, although this is most common with penicillin. Immediate (IgE-mediated) or delayed hypersensitivity may occur, the latter resulting in serum sickness, erythema multiforme, lupus syndrome or haemolytic anaemia.

The penicillins and cephalosporins are the safest antibiotics to use in pregnancy. They cross the placenta (fetal levels are 70% of those in the mother) and are therefore effective against fetal infections such as congenital syphilis. Rifampicin, the tetracyclines, the sulphonamides and trimethoprim (co-trimoxazole) have all been associated with fetal abnormalities. If given late in pregnancy, sulphonamides may precipitate kernicterus (by displacement of bilirubin from albumin). The tetracyclines cross the placenta and can damage bone and stain developing teeth. Streptomycin can cause 8th nerve damage in the fetus.

Antiviral agents

Because of the intracellular nature of viral infection, there are few effective antiviral agents. The very limited group of such materials includes:

1. Amantadine (an anti-Parkinsonian agent), which is effective against influenza.

2. Idoxuridine, cytosine arabinoside and adenine arabinoside, which impair viral nucleic acid synthesis by competitive inhibition of enzymes and are active against herpes. Systemic administration has toxic effects on bone marrow and is only used in severe herpetic encephalitis. Topical application of idoxuridine has been used in herpetic conjunctivitis and other mucocutaneous lesions.

3. Acyclovir, which is highly active against herpes but does not prevent recurrence. It may be administered systemically or locally.

4. Inosine pranobex, which enhances T cell response to many viruses, including herpes and HIV.

5. Interferons, which have been used as topical applications to speed resolution of herpes lesions.

6. Zidovudine, which is active against HIV by competing with thymidine in the process in which viral RNA is converted into viral DNA by reverse transcriptase. The drug cannot eliminate the primary virus, but does reduce HIV-related mortality rate and the incidence and severity of opportunistic infections.

Table 7.8. Summary of antibiotic pharmacology

Class	Examples	Route of administration	Spectrum of activity	Side-effects	Other observations
Penicillins (based on 6-amino-penicillanic acid)	Benzylpenicillin (crystapen)	Parenteral	Streptococci, staphylococci, Neisseria, Pneumococcus, Clostridium, Treponema pallidum, Corynebacterium, anthrax, Actinomyces	Allergy, convulsions after massive i.v. bolus	This is the most powerful penicillin and is the drug of choice for sensitive organisms. Inactivated by lactamase
	Phenoxymethyl-penicillin (penicillin V)	Oral	As above but absorption inadequate for serious infections. Used for rheumatic fever prophylaxis	Allergy	
	Ampicillin and amoxycillin	Oral and parenteral	As above and many Gram-negative infections	Allergy. Rash in patients with infectious mononucleosis	Is inactivated by lactamase. Amoxycillin is absorbed twice as well as ampicillin. Excreted in bile and urine
	Cloxacillin (Orbenin)	Oral and parenteral	Gram-positives only, but stable to lactamase	Allergy	Highly protein bound. Flucloxacillin is better absorbed
	Carbenicillin (Pyopen)	Parenteral only (preferably intravenous)	Gram-positives and negatives, but in particular Pseudomonas	Allergy	Pseudomonas infection probably only indication. Large doses (up to 24 g/day) required
Cephalo-sporins (based on 7-amino-ceph-alosporic acid)	a) 1st generation: Cephaloridine Cephalothin			Allergy (about 10% who have penicillin allergies will also react to cephalosporins). Cephaloridine can cause dose-related tubular necrosis, especially in conjunction with lasix	
	Cefuroxime Cephazolin	Parenteral	Broad spectrum but inactive against Bacteroides, Strep. faecalis, Pseudomonas		
	Cephalexin	Oral			
	Cephradine	Oral and parenteral			
	b) 2nd generation: Cefoxitin Cephamycins	Parenteral	Broad spectrum; stable to β-lactamase	Allergy	

Table 7.8. (*continued*)

Class	Examples	Route of administration	Spectrum of activity	Side-effects	Other observations
Aminoglycosides	Streptomycin Neomycin Kanamycin Gentamicin Tobramycin	Not orally absorbed but may be given to reduce intestinal bacterial load	Broad spectrum but inactive against anaerobes. Many resistant strains emerging	Ototoxic and nephrotoxic. Drug fever. Potentiate neuromuscular blocking drugs	Streptomycin now reserved for treatment of tuberculosis, because resistant strains develop rapidly. Avoid in pregnancy
Tetracyclines	Oxytetracycline Doxycycline	Oral or parenteral depending on type used	Broad spectrum but specially indicated for brucellosis, chlamydial and rickettsial infections	Damage developing bones and teeth. Photosensitivity	Bacteriostatic
Lincosamines	Lincomycin Clindamycin	Oral or parenteral	Broad but indicated for *Staph. aureus* and *Bacteroides*	Pseudomembranous colitis	Concentrated in bone, therefore useful for osteomyelitis
Sulphonamides	a) Single agent Sulphamezathine Sulphadiazine	Oral	Broad spectrum. Very active against streptococci, pneumococci and *Neisseria*. Relatively inactive against *Staphylococcus*. Resistance common	Older insoluble compounds caused crystal formation in kidney. Erythema multiforme	Displace bilirubin from albumin binding site, thereby aggravating neonatal jaundice
	b) Combined with trimethoprim in co-trimoxazole	Oral or intravenous, not intramuscular			
Erythromycin	Estolate Stearate	Oral (estolate better absorbed)	Similar to benzylpenicillin including *Haemophilus*. Drug of choice for pertussis prophylaxis	Cholestatic jaundice, particularly with the estolate	Excretion in bile

Table 7.8. *(continued)*

Class	Examples	Route of administration	Spectrum of activity	Side-effects	Other observations
Chloram-phenicol	Chloromycetin	Oral or in-travenous. Not. intra-muscular	Broad, but used for typhoid and haemophilus meningitis	Aplastic anaemia	Causes 'grey' babies when given to infants but does not harm fetus. Bacteriostatic
Metronidazole	Flagyl	Oral or intravenous	*Trichomonas, Giardia,* amoebae and many bacteria, especially *Bacteroides*	Stomatitis	Should not be given with alcohol (and may promote fetal alcohol syndrome in pregnancy)
Quinolones	Ciprofloxacin	Oral or intravenous	Broad, especially for Gram-negative organisms		Unlikely to cause resistance
Nitrofurantoin		Oral	Broad spectrum, widely used for urinary tract infections	Pulmonary infiltration	Lack of R-factor resistance

Antifungal agents

The polyenes (nystatin) and imidazoles (clotrimazole, ketoconazole) are specific antifungal agents used topically for vaginal infections. Ketoconazole inhibits desmolase activity (see Fig. 4.6a) with a reduction in androstenedione and testosterone and an increase in progesterone and 17-hydroxyprogesterone levels.

Antimalarial agents

Chloroquine (orally or by injection) is the drug of choice for benign tertian malaria (*Plasmodium vivax, P. ovale, P. malariae*). Many strains of *P. falciparum* are resistant (malignant tertian malaria). Chloroquine can cause gastrointestinal disturbances, psychotic episodes and convulsions, and corneal and retinal damage. Prophylactic doses of chloroquine do not damage the fetal eye.

Pharmacology of sex steroids

The 'combined' oral contraceptive pill contains an oestrogen and a progestogen, whereas the so-called mini-pills contain only a progestogen. The former inhibit ovulation; the latter rely on peripheral changes for their contraceptive effect. Larger doses of progestational compounds will, however, prevent ovulation, and this effect is seen with Depo-provera (medroxyprogesterone acetate injections).

Oestrogens

Oestradiol is broken down in the stomach, but an ethinyl group at the 17 position confers oral activity. Ethinyloestradiol is the most widely used oestrogen in oral contraceptives. The other oestrogen sometimes used is the 3-methyl ester of ethinyloestradiol, mestranol (Fig. 7.1), which has half the potency of ethinyloestradiol.

Other orally active oestrogens are sometimes used therapeutically (e.g. for menopausal symptoms):

1. *Premarin*: conjugated oestrone from the urine of pregnant mares
2. *Oestradiol valerate*: converted to oestrone during absorption
3. *Oestradiol*: on a micronised solid phase, also converted to oestrone during absorption

The side-effects of oestrogens include vascular complications, particularly deep vein thrombosis. Liver adenomas are more common, and other side-effects include hypertension, cholecystitis, headaches, migraine, weight gain, depression and altered libido. Biochemical effects include an increase in high-density lipoprotein cholesterol (HDL-C), an increase in triglycerides, impaired glucose tolerance and increased thyroxine and cortisol binding.

The efficacy of oestrogen-containing contraceptive agents may be reduced by concomitant administration of antibiotic, especially rifampicin and griseofulvin.

Progestogens

Progestogenic drugs, like progesterone itself, have little effect without oestrogen. The potency of the different progestogens has been measured by their ability to delay menstruation (the Greenblatt test), although this correlates poorly with other measures, such as contraceptive potency. Progesterone itself is destroyed by stomach acid but can be administered as a suppository. There are three forms of progesterone which are absorbed after oral administration:

1. Dydrogesterone (6-dehydro-*retro*-progesterone) (Fig. 7.2), which is a very weak progestogen.

2. 17α-Hydroxyprogesterone derivatives (Fig. 7.3), the best known of which is medroxyprogesterone acetate (Fig. 7.3). An injection (150 mg) of this substance lasts at least 3 months and acts by inhibiting luteinising hormone release. Other 17-OH derivatives are megestrol acetate and chlormadinone acetate.

3. 19-nor-Progesterones: the commonest progestogen in oral contraceptives. Removal of the CH_3 group from the 19 position of testosterone protects the steroid from acid breakdown. The 19-nor-progesterones are related to this compound and all have some residual androgenic activity. Norgestrel (Fig. 7.2) is the most potent and widely used; it is made synthetically. Unlike the other widely used norsteroids (norethisterone, ethynodiol diacetate and lynoestrenol), it is not partly metabolised to oestrogen. Three newer progestogens, norgestimate, desogestrel and gestodene

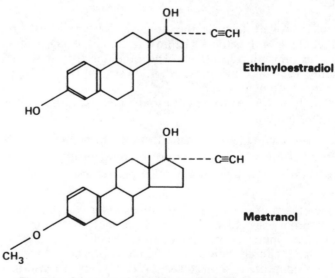

Fig. 7.1. Structures of ethinyloestradiol and mestranol.

are all chemically related to levonorgestrel. Cycle control is improved with a lower incidence of intermenstrual bleeding and less adverse effects on blood lipids. Norgestimate and desogestrel have to be transformed into metabolites for their biological activity and are of similar potency to levonorgestrel. Gestodene is active in native form and is twice as potent as norgestrel. Gestodene has anti-oestrogenic activity and low androgenic activity.

Side-effects of progestogens such as headache, breast discomfort and weight gain are difficult to separate from those of oestrogen. Breakthrough bleeding is an important side-effect of progestogen-only contraceptives and dry vagina, reduced libido and dizziness have been attributed to this therapy. Progestogens suppress HDL-C and increase LDL-C.

Progestogens are also used to treat dysfunctional uterine bleeding, dysmenorrhoea, endometriosis and endometrial cancer. They are not useful in habitual or threatened abortion, and the 19-norsteroids, because of their androgenic effect, are contraindicated in this condition.

Antiprogesterones

These either inhibit progesterone formation (11β-dehydrogenase antagonists, which may also inhibit cortisol secretion) or block the receptor (mifepristone; RU 486). They are abortifacient and contraceptive.

Anti-androgens

Anti-androgens include cyproterone, spironolactone, megestrol acetate, medrogesterone, stilboestrol, flutamide and cimetidine. Cyproterone acetate acts

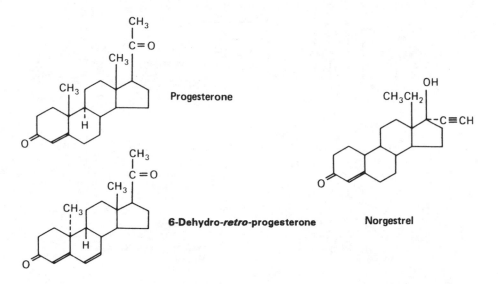

Fig. 7.2. Structures of progesterone, 6-dehydro-*retro*-progesterone and norgestrel.

by suppressing both testosterone and LH production, and competes with testosterone for target hormone receptors. It is used for hypersexuality in males, and severe hirsutism in females. Side-effects include adrenocortical suppression.

Anti-oestrogens

Oestradiol synthesis can be blocked by the aromatase inhibitor testolactone.

Androgens

Oral testosterone is ineffective because the steroid is rapidly inactivated in the gut wall and liver. For male hypogonadism, testosterone esters are given by intramuscular injection or subcutaneous implantation, or more recently by oral administration of testosterone undecanoate dissolved in oleic acid.

Antithyroid drugs

Carbimazole and propylthiouracil act by interfering with synthesis of thyroid hormones. Both can cross the placenta or enter breast milk, and in high doses may cause fetal or infant goitre and hypothyroidism. Rarely, carbimazole causes aplasia cutis of the neonate.

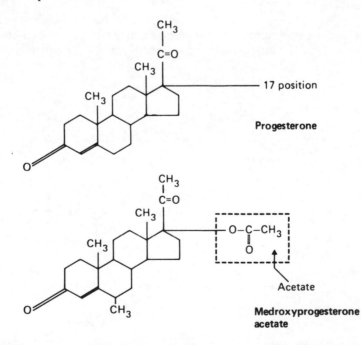

Fig. 7.3. The 17 position of the progesterone molecule and one of the 17α-hydroxyprogesterone derivatives, medroxyprogesterone acetate.

Drugs affecting contraction of the uterus

Mechanism of myometrial contraction

The myometrial cell contains myofibrils of actin and myosin. Under the influence of myosin light chain kinase, the actin and myosin slide on each other to produce a contraction. The reaction is triggered by a complex of a peptide (calmodulin) and calcium. Hormones that affect uterine activity bind to surface receptors and activate phospholipase C. This hydrolyses phosphatidyl 4,5-biphosphate to diacylglycerol and inositol triphosphate. The latter leads to release of calcium from intracellular storage areas and its intake from the extracellular space via membrane-based calcium channels (so-called slow channels, as opposed to fast channels through which sodium enters the cell during depolarisation).

Drugs causing uterine contractions

Oxytocin

Oxytocin (see Chapter 4) acts via specific receptors on the myometrial cell membrane; the number of these receptors is under control of oestrogens and increases progressively during pregnancy. At term the dose required to induce labour is 0.5–15 mU/min. The appropriate dose produces regular contractions with a normal resting intrauterine pressure of 8–12 mmHg. Hyperstimulation results in a progressively raised resting pressure (hypertonus). This occludes the placental circulation and may result in uterine rupture and amniotic fluid embolus.

Oxytocin has 5% of the antidiuretic effect of vasopressin (ADH). Hyponatraemia and water intoxication may occur when high doses are administered with large amounts of fluid. Fetal hyponatraemia and neonatal jaundice have also been attributed to oxytocin administration

Ergometrine

Ergometrine produces a prolonged tonic contraction of the uterus with superimposed rapid clonic contractions. The action takes 7 min to begin after intramuscular injection and 45 s after intravenous injection.

In women who are already hypertensive, a transient but considerable increase in blood pressure may follow intravenous ergometrine. It may also cause vomiting and should be avoided during Caesarean section under epidural analgesia.

Prostaglandins

Prostaglandins are based on a 20-carbon parent compound, prostanoic acid (Fig. 7.4). The four classic groups (A, B, E and F) are classified according

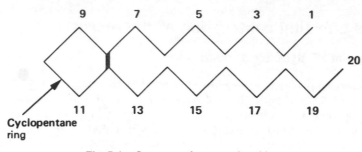

Fig. 7.4.   Structure of prostanoic acid.

to the structure of the cyclopentane ring; the number of double bonds in the side-chain is indicated by a subscript numeral after the latter (PGE_1 has one double bond, PGE_2 has two).

Prostaglandins are synthesised from arachidonic acid; this is hydrolysed by prostaglandin synthetase (cyclo-oxygenase) to form the precursor cyclic endoperoxides. Three types of prostaglandins are manufactured – the four classic groups above, thromboxanes and prostacyclins. Prostacyclin is synthesised mainly in the walls of the blood vessels; thromboxane is synthesised in vessel walls and platelets. Prostacylin causes smooth muscle relaxation and inhibits platelet aggregation, whereas thromboxane A_2 has the reverse effects. Thromboxane A_2 has a 6-membered oxane ring in place of the cyclopentane ring.

Prostacyclin and thromboxane production increases in pregnancy, sources including placenta, membranes and decidua. Platelet cyclo-oxygenase is about 20 times as sensitive to antiprostaglandins, such as aspirin, as the vessel wall enzyme. For this reason *low doses* of these agents increase the ratio of prostacyclin to thromboxane in the spiral arteries during pregnancy. Labetalol (an α- and β-blocking antihypertensive agent) also enhances the prostacyclin to thromboxane ratio. The latter effect may be independent of α- or β-receptor effect. Calcium channel blocking agents also inhibit platelet aggregation by enhancing the effects of prostacyclin.

All prostaglandins act and are metabolised at local level. Prostaglandins that enter the circulation are rapidly inactivated by pulmonary enzymes.

Prostaglandin $F_{2\alpha}$ causes contraction of both the pregnant and the non-pregnant uterus. Prostaglandin E_2 has the same effect in vivo (at 10 times the potency), but in vitro or when instilled directly into the non-pregnant uterus it causes relaxation. Prostaglandins have many other effects. They are necessary for ovum release, luteolysis in many species, and maintenance of the fetal pattern of circulation. The umbilical arteries are the richest source of prostacyclin, and both prostacyclin and PGE_2 are secreted in the wall of the ductus arteriosus and maintain its patency. The secretory endometrium produces large amounts of prostaglandin $F_{2\alpha}$.

Labour and abortion may be induced by systemic or local use of PGE_2 or $PGF_{2\alpha}$. Systemic administration produces severe gastrointestinal symptoms and more rarely causes bronchospasm and hypotension or hypertension. Local administration may be intra-amniotic, extra-amniotic or vaginal. The principal action by the vaginal route is to induce cervical ripening by stimulating collagenase production and glycosaminoglycan secretion from fibroblasts. Intra-amniotic prostaglandins cause prolonged uterine spasm and may result in cervical laceration. Inadvertent injection into the myometrium produces severe tissue necrosis.

Agents acting on adrenergic receptors

The uterus has both α-excitatory and β-inhibitory receptors. β-Blockers (propranolol) will enhance uterine activity in late pregnancy.

Drugs that relax the uterus (tocolytics)

β-Adrenergic receptor stimulants

β_1-Receptors are responsible for actions such as increases of heart rate, lipolysis and relaxation of intestinal smooth muscle; β_2-receptors mediate glycogenolysis and smooth muscle relaxation. Earlier β-agonists (e.g. isoxsuprine) had both β_1 and β_2 activity. Later products have relatively more β_2 effect and thus provide a greater degree of uterine relaxation for a given increase in heart rate. Drugs in this class include ritodrine, orciprenaline, salbutamol, terbutaline and fenoterol. β-Agonists promote lung surfactant production and increase uterine blood-flow by abolishing uterine contractions, increasing cardiac output and exerting a vasodilator effect. The more lipid-soluble agents, such as ritodrine, cross the placenta and have a direct stimulant effect on the fetal heart. β-Agonists down-regulate their own receptors; thus a progressively higher dosage may be required to produce an equivalent effect.

Side-effects include tachycardia (and, in very large doses, hypotension and arrhythmias), hyperglycaemia and hyperinsulinaemia, tremor, palpitations, sweating and headache. Severe heart disease, thyrotoxicosis, uncontrolled diabetes and treatment with monoamine oxidase inhibitors are contraindications to the use of β-agonists.

Beta-stimulant therapy is often combined with large doses of glucocorticoids to promote fetal lung maturity. This may further aggravate hyperglycaemia and may, in rare cases, cause pulmonary oedema.

Aminophylline

Aminophylline relaxes the myometrium by inhibiting phosphodiesterase and thus the degradation of intracellular cAMP.

Antiprostaglandins

Prostaglandin synthetase inhibitors such as indomethacin and flufenamic acid are potent tocolytics. They may cause premature closure of the ductus arteriosus and pulmonary hypertension. Indomethacin and aspirin, unlike flufenamic acid, irreversibly alter prostaglandin synthetase. Platelets have

Table 7.9. Alkylating agents

Agent	Feature
Mustine (nitrogen mustard)	Used in Hodgkin's disease. Very irritant to tissues (given into tubing of fast-running infusion). Severe nausea
Cyclophosphamide (Endoxana)	Used in non-Hodgkin's lymphoma and solid tumours. Is active until metabolised in liver. Can cause haemorrhagic cystitis
Melphalan (Alkeran)	Used in myeloma and as local infusion for melanoma. Marrow toxicity is delayed
Busulphan (Myleran)	Used in chronic myeloid leukaemia. Can cause pulmonary fibrosis
Thiotepa	Used in solid tumours

+ CHLORAMBUCIL

no nucleus and cannot resynthesise this enzyme. *Low doses* of aspirin and indomethacin therefore have a more marked effect on platelets than on other tissues, such as vessel endothelium.

Other tocolytic agents

These include:

1. Halothane

2. Ethanol (by inhibition of oxytocin release)

3. Calcium antagonists such as nifedipine (these decrease the size of calcium channels; oxytocin increases the size)

4. Diazoxide

5. Magnesium sulphate

6. Papaverine

7. Phentolamine (α-receptor blocker)

Anticancer drugs (cytotoxic agents)

These drugs interfere with cell division and thus affect any dividing cell, be it normal or neoplastic. Their effects on tumour cells are almost always associated with severe side-effects, including: (a) bone marrow and gastro-intestinal damage, (b) opportunistic infection, (c) alopecia and dermatitis, (d) interruption of spermatogenesis and premature menopause, (e) fetal damage, (f) an increased incidence of leukaemia, and (g) toxic reaction to destruction of large tumour masses. Because of their effects on the reticuloendothelial system, certain cytotoxics are used as immunosuppressive agents.

Anti-cancer drugs include:

1. *Alkylating agents* (Table 7.9): These cause structural damage to chromosomes at the time of replication during interphase.

2. *Platinum derivatives*: These cause cross-linkage of complementary DNA strands, thus preventing replication. Agents such as *cis*-dichlorodiamine platinum are used for solid tumours (e.g. ovarian cancer). They are

Table 7.10. Antimetabolites

Class	Mechanism of action	Indications	Remarks
Folic acid antagonists (methotrexate)	Inhibits folic reductase. Does not cross blood–brain barrier	Choriocarcinoma, Burkitt's lymphoma, acute leukaemia	Toxic and teratogenic action on embryonic mesenchyme. Orally absorbed
Antipurines (mercaptopurine, azothioprine)	Chemically related to adenine and hypoxanthine (azothioprine is converted to mercaptopurine in the liver)	Acute leukaemia (mercaptopurine) Immunosuppression (azothioprine)	May cause jaundice Allopurinol enhances activity
Antipyrimidines (fluorouracil (5-FU), cytosine arabinoside)	Prevents normal pyrimidine insertion into DNA	Gastrointestinal cancers and herpes infections (5-FU). Acute leukaemia (cytosine arabinoside)	

nephrotoxic and ototoxic, but high doses can be administered if followed by osmotic diuresis.

3. *Antimetabolites* (Table 7.10): These simulate natural substrates and block normal metabolic pathways.

4. *Spindle poisons* (vincristine and vinblastine): Like colchicine, these plant alkaloids bind to tubulin and cause metaphase arrest by interfering with microtubular assembly. In addition to the usual side-effects, they may cause cranial nerve palsies.

5. *Antibiotics*, e.g. actinomycin D, daunorubicin, doxorubicin (adriamycin) and mitozantrone: These interfere with RNA replication. They can cause severe alopecia, supraventricular tachycardia and cardiomyopathy, and because of their irritant effects must be given intravenously. Bleomycin is relatively free of bone marrow toxicity, but causes pulmonary fibrosis. It is particularly active in squamous carcinomas.

6. *Steroids*: Sex steroids are sometimes used in the treatment of target organ malignancies (e.g. progesterone for carcinoma of the endometrium and kidney; corticosteroids and androgens for premenopausal breast cancer; oestrogens for postmenopausal breast cancer).

7. *Radioactive agents*: A number of radioactive agents have been used for their effects on specific tumours. These include: (a) ^{32}P (β emission, half-life 14 days), instilled into the peritoneal cavity for malignant ascites; (b) ^{131}I (β and γ emission, half-life 8 days), used for thyroid ablation; and (c) ^{198}Au (radiogold, β and γ emission, half-life 1.5 days), used in malignant effusions.

8. *Interferons*: These have been used with some success in the treatment of hairy cell leukaemia, chronic myelogenous leukaemia, some lymphomas, melanoma, renal carcinoma and myeloma.

General anaesthetic agents

The usual procedure for general anaesthesia is administration of a premedication (Table 7.11), induction with an intravenous agent (Table 7.12) and maintenance with an inhalational agent (Table 7.13), together with, where appropriate, a muscle relaxant (Table 7.14). Most anaesthetic agents are lipid-soluble and cross the placenta freely; the exception is the muscle relaxants, which are highly ionised and are therefore not transferred to the fetus.

Local anaesthetic agents

Local anaesthetics cause a reversible block to nerve conduction. They are basic drugs, and neuronal uptake is inhibited in tissues with a low pH (e.g. around abscess cavities). Pain fibres and autonomic fibres are more sensitive than touch, temperature and motor fibres. Although the action is local, the

Table 7.11. Features of commonly used premedication agents

Agent	Features
Anticholinergic agents (atropine, hyoscine)	Dry bronchial and salivary secretions. Prevent excess bradycardia and hypotension with agents such as halothane. Can cause fetal tachycardia
Narcotic analgesics (morphine, papaveretum, pethidine)	Facilitate induction and alleviate anxiety. Provide additional analgesia during and after surgery. May depress respiration
Benzodiazepines (diazepam, lorazepam)	Anxiolytic and sedative
Phenothiazines (promethazine, chlorpromazine)	Anxiolytic and anti-emetic. May depress respiration

Table 7.12. Features of intravenous anaesthetics. All act in one arm–brain circulation time (10–30 s)

Agent	Features
Thiopentone sodium	Damages subcutaneous tissues. Avoid with porphyria. Recovery slow and effects may persist for 6–8 h
Methohexitone sodium	Induction less smooth than with thiopentone but recovery is more rapid
Ketamine	Can be given by intramuscular injection. In adults can cause hallucinations and psychotic sequelae. Increases muscle tone and therefore not compatible with muscle relaxants. Causes severe transient hypertension
Diazepam	Delay of 3 min for effect; dose varies greatly between patients

Table 7.13. Features of inhalational anaesthetics. (Though usually for maintenance, inhalational anaesthetics can also be used for induction)

Agent	Features
Nitrous oxide	Weak but markedly analgesic, acts in 2–3 min. Concentration 70%–75% with 20% oxygen during induction and 30% during maintenance. An additional volatile agent is essential for complete anaesthesia. Widely used as an analgesic in obstetrics (Entonox: 50% N$_2$O/50% O$_2$)
Halothane	Most widely used maintenance agent. Non-irritant, promotes muscle relaxation (including uterus), rapid recovery. Causes hypotension. Repeated use can lead to liver damage
Trichloroethylene	Weak but markedly analgesic. Used in subanaesthetic doses (0.35%–0.5%) in obstetrics. Recovery may be prolonged (vomiting)
Ether	Inflammable, irritant, high incidence of vomiting and bronchoconstriction. Little used

Table 7.14. Agents used for muscle relaxation during surgery (neuromuscular blocking agents). The first three agents are 'non-depolarising' and their action may be reversed by cholinesterase inhibitors (e.g. neostigmine)

Agent	Features
Tubocurarine	Competes with acetylcholine for the receptor site at the neuromuscular junction. Acts in 3–5 min and lasts for 30 min. Can cause histamine release, with rash and hypotension; should be avoided in myasthenia gravis
Pancuronium	As tubocurarine, but faster action and no histamine release
Gallamine	More rapid than either of above, but causes tachycardia
Suxamethonium	Acts like acetylcholine at neuromuscular junction, but depolarisation is prolonged because of slow breakdown. The action is rapid and lasts for 5 min. Paralysis is preceded by muscle fasciculation; sharp rise in plasma K$^+$ and creatine phosphokinase. Prolonged paralysis may occur in patients with low or atypical plasma pseudocholinesterase. There is no antagonist

side-effects (convulsive excitation of the central nervous system followed by depression; hypotension) are the result of systemic absorption. All local anaesthetics cross the placenta, and umbilical blood concentrations are 40%–70% of those in the mother. Most local anaesthetics cause vasodilatation, and they are often combined with adrenaline (1:80000 to 1:200000; maximum 500 µg). Adrenaline should be avoided in patients taking tricyclic antidepressants.

Commonly used local anaesthetic agents are shown in Table 7.15.

Drugs of abuse

Cocaine can produce a rise in maternal blood pressure, a decrease in uterine blood-flow, fetal hypoxia, placental abruption and neonatal addiction.

Table 7.15.   Features of commonly used local anaesthetics

Agent	Features
Lignocaine	Acts rapidly, effects (with adrenaline) last 1.5 h. Destroyed in the liver
Bupivacaine	Acts slowly (30 min) but lasts up to 8 h. Commonly used for epidural analgesia (duration 2–3 h; maximum dose 150 mg/4 h). It is highly protein bound, thereby limiting transplacental exchange
Mepivacaine	Slightly longer acting than lignocaine; used in spinal anaesthesia. Does not cause vasodilatation
Prilocaine	Similar to lignocaine
Benzocaine	Weak agent used for surface analgesia in mouth and anus
Amethocaine, cinchocaine, cocaine, procaine	All have side-effects or other disadvantages and are replaced by agents named above

General aspects of pharmacology in pregnancy

The potential for teratogenic effects explains the extreme caution that must be exercised in prescribing during pregnancy (Table 7.16). In addition, the following general factors may influence the choice of drug or route of administration:

1. Gastric emptying time is increased so that orally administered drugs may be very slowly absorbed, especially during labour.

2. Intestinal motility is reduced, which may enhance overall absorption.

3. Total body water is increased by as much as 8 litres.

4. Plasma albumin is reduced by as much as 10 g/litre. Therefore plasma binding of drugs is decreased.

5. Fat stores are increased and act as a reservoir for lipid-soluble drugs.

6. Liver metabolism increases but not liver blood-flow. Drugs whose elimination depends on liver enzymes can show large increases in clearance during pregnancy, e.g. phenytoin and theophylline. Drugs which are eliminated at a rate mainly dependent on liver blood-flow, such as propranolol, show no change in clearance.

7. Increased renal plasma flow and glomerular filtration rate will increase renal clearance of water-soluble drugs (an important factor with lithium, digoxin, pancuronium and antibiotics such as ampicillin, cephalosporins and aminoglycosides).

8. The half-life of more lipid-soluble drugs may increase during pregnancy, whereas the reverse may be true for less lipid-soluble drugs.

9. The human placenta can metabolise drugs and thus contribute to their clearance.

10. Lipid-soluble substances up to a molecular weight of 600–1000 can readily cross the placenta. Water-soluble substances cross only up to a molecular weight of 100. In general, drugs that cross the blood–brain barrier and affect the central nervous system will also cross the placenta.

Table 7.16. Some examples of teratogenic agents. The effects vary according to the state of pregnancy. At days 0–17 (postfertilisation) the embryo dies and aborts. At days 18–55, the time of organogenesis, teratogenic effects occur. At days 56–term differentiation is not affected but development may be (e.g. microcephaly due to drugs and toxins)

Agent	Effects
Thalidomide	Multiple, especially limb defects
Cytotoxic drugs[a]	Multiple
Irradiation	Leukaemia, carcinoma of the thyroid
Alcohol	Fetal alcohol syndrome
Phenytoin[b]	Cleft palate, cardiac anomalies, minor skeletal defects
Warfarin	Nasal hypoplasia, chondrodysplasia punctata. CNS abnormalities
Lithium	Cardiac anomalies
Quinine	Hypoplasia of optic nerves and congenital deafness
Diethylstilboestrol	Carcinoma of vagina in young women, vaginal adenosis
Cyproterone acetate and possibly 19-norsteroids	Androgenise female fetus
Aminoglycosides	Deafness
Tetracycline	Bone abnormalities
Glucocorticoids	Cleft lip
Maternal hyperthermia	CNS abnormalities
Iodine	Congenital hypothyroidism
Pseudoephedrine	Gastroschisis
Isotretinoin	Hypoplastic ears, malformation of facial bones, cardiac defects, thymic aplasia, hydrocephalus

[a] Especially folic acid antagonists and alkylating agents.
[b] Probably due to effects on folate metabolism.

11. Placental transfer of drugs is also related to protein binding in maternal blood (only the unbound fraction is freely diffusible).

12. In general, if a drug can be absorbed orally it will also cross the placenta.

13. The fetus is no more sensitive than the adult to carcinogenic agents (as opposed to teratogenic agents).

General aspects of pharmacology during breast feeding

Three categories of drug cross into breast milk:

1. Drugs that are undetectable in the baby, including warfarin, which is bound to maternal proteins, and aminoglycosides, which are not absorbed from the gut.

2. Drugs that reach the infant, but in insignificant amounts, e.g. non-narcotic

Table 7.17. Drugs for which deleterious effects during lactation
have been reported

Amantadine	Carbimazole	Lithium
Amiodarone	Cascara	Phenindione
Anthraquinone	Chloramphenicol	Primidone
Antineoplastics	Ephedrine	Radioactive agents
Atropine	Ergotamine	Streptomycin
Barbiturates	Iodine	Sulphonamides
Benzodiazepines	Kanamycin	Thiouracil
Bromides		

analgesics, penicillin and cephalosporin antibiotics, and antihypertensive
drugs. Oral contraceptives with low doses of oestrogen do not suppress
established lactation and are not harmful to the baby.

3. Drugs that reach the infant in doses sufficient to cause harm, e.g.
laxatives, barbiturates, lithium, cytotoxics and immunosuppressive drugs.
Drugs for which specific deleterious effects have been reported are shown in
Table 7.17.

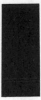

Appendix A

Statistics

The following terms are commonly used in the description and comparison of numerical data in biomedicine:

Mean (arithmetic mean): obtained by adding the observed values and dividing by the total number of values. If the values are normally distributed (i.e. give a bell-shaped Gaussian curve), the mean is the same as the median and the mode (see below)

Mode: the most frequently occurring value

Median: the value above which half the observations lie and below which the other half lie (note: in non-normal distributions the mean, median and mode may be different values)

Standard deviation (s.d.) (root mean square deviation): a measure of the dispersion of a set of values. The mean ±2 s.d. embraces 95% of a normally distributed (Gaussian) population

Standard error of the mean (s.e.m.): s.d. divided by $\sqrt{n}$ or $\sqrt{(n-1)}$. An estimate of the limits to the mean of the total population from which the sample observations were drawn

Variance (mean square variance): the square of the s.d.

Centiles (or percentiles): e.g. 10th centile is the value below which 10% of the population lies and above which 90% of the population lies

Null hypothesis: hypothesis that there is no difference between two sets of data

Probability P: frequency with which an event would occur at random, given a total frequency of 1. Thus P of 0.05 indicates that an event would occur 1 in 20 times at random. P of 0.05 is traditionally used as the cut-off point for 'statistical significance': figures of 0.05 or below are thus considered non-random

Student's t test: the standard test for comparing the difference between two means

Chi-squared test (χ^2): the standard method for comparing distributions, e.g. between the observed and expected frequency of a given event

F test: the standard method for comparing the size of variances

Correlation: the relation between two variables

Linear regression: the standard method for determining whether two variables are correlated (e.g. if $x = y$ and $2x = 2y$, x and y are correlated)

Coefficient of correlation (r) (regression coefficient): indicates the degree of correlation between x and y. A value of 1 is perfect correlation, a value of 0 is no correlation at all

Prevalence: number of patients in the whole population (e.g. per 100 000) who have the disease at the time of the study

Incidence: number of patients who develop the disease in a given period of time (e.g. 1 year)

In addition, the following terms are frequently used in obstetric epidemiology:

Stillbirth and stillbirth rate: a stillbirth is a baby born after 24 weeks gestation showing no signs of life. The stillbirth rate is the number of stillbirths per 1000 total (live and still) births

Neonatal death (NND) and neonatal death rate: neonatal death is death within 28 days of birth. 'Early' NNDs are those occurring within 7 days (first week deaths). The neonatal death rate is the number of NNDs per 1000 live births

Infant mortality rate: number of infants dying during the first year per 1000 live births

Perinatal mortality rate: number of stillbirths and first week deaths per 1000 total births

Parity: number of previous pregnancies completed after 28 weeks

Gravidity: number of all pregnancies ending at any gestation, including any current pregnancy

Statistics defining 'test' performance:

Sensitivity: the ability of the test to include patients it is designed to include. It is the probability of the test being positive in patients with the condition. It is calculated as: true-positive/(true-positive + false-negative)

Specificity: the ability of the test to exclude patients it is designed to exclude. It is the probability of a negative test given absence of the condition. It is calculated as: true-negative/(true-negative + false-positive)

Predictive value positive: the probability of having the condition if the test is positive. Calculated as: true-positive/(true-positive + false-positive)

Likelihood ratio: calculated as sensitivity/(1 − specificity)

Appendix B

Ultrasound

Audible sound has a frequency of 16–16 000 cycles per second (cps). Medical ultrasound uses a range of 1 million to 10 million cps (1–10 MHz); 3.5 MHz is most commonly used in obstetrics. These frequencies are produced by the effect of an electrical current on a 'crystal' made from a synthetic ceramic ('piezoelectric effect'). The crystal is shaped to produce a focused beam of ultrasound. The beam is delivered as a series of pulses (usually approx. 1 m/s). Echoes from interfaces between tissues of different densities return to the crystal and are converted back to an electrical pulse. The wavelength determines the axial resolution of the system (typically 1 mm), while beam width largely determines lateral resolution (3–10 mm according to depth). The velocity of sound in soft tissue is 1540 m/s (air 330 m/s; bone 4000 m/s). Attenuation of the sound beam increases linearly with frequency.

Procedures for signal processing are summarised in Table B.1. Display systems include cathode ray tubes (oscilloscope) and analogue or digital scan converters (TV/video format). Real-time scanners are of four types described in Table B.2.

Table B.1. Terms commonly used in describing signal processing in ultrasound systems

Term	Meaning
A-mode (amplitude modulation)	Echo displayed as blip or deflection on oscilloscope. Size related to strength of echo
B-mode (brightness modulation)	Movements of transducer yield a series of dots which build a two-dimensional image
Real-time	Transducer moved automatically (mechanical or electronic) to generate successive B-scans (typically 15–60 frames per second)
M-mode (time-position mode)	B-scan displayed continuously with respect to time (i.e. demonstrates movements)
Grey-scale	Selective amplification of low-level echoes from soft tissues

Table B.2.   Types of real-time scanner

Type	Principle
Mechanical linear array	A single transducer is moved to and fro at high speed
Electronic linear array	A line of multiple transducers (64) is activated sequentially
Mechanical sector scanner	Transducer element rocked mechanically in a sector ranging from 15° to 90°
Electronic sector scanner (phased arrays)	Group of transducers activated sequentially to produce a sector beam

Doppler ultrasound systems can be used to study blood flow velocity. The systems are continuous wave (CW) or pulsed wave (PW). CW systems are small and cheap but have poor resolution. PW systems can determine the depth from which signals are gathered. They are often combined with imaging systems as duplex scanners, or with real-time imaging systems to provide colour flow mapping (flow is indicated by red in one direction, blue in the other).

Index